Human

An Operator's Manual

Human

An Operator's Manual

by

Chris Douglas, M.A.

Elliott Douglas Publishing

Human: An Operator's Manual
by Chris Douglas, M.A.

First published in Canada in 2010 by
Elliott Douglas Publishing
Suite 506 4058 Lakeshore Road,
Kelowna, B.C.
V1W 1V6
www.elliottdouglas.com

Cover design and illustrations: Mishell Raedeke
Interior design: Jill Veitch

Canada Cataloguing in Publication Data

Douglas, Chris, 1975-
Human : an operator's manual / Chris Douglas.

ISBN 978-0-9865717-1-8

1. Health--Popular works. 2. Body, Human--Popular works.
3. Self-actualization (Psychology). I. Title.

RA776.D69 2010   613   C2010-905124-6

Printed and bound in Canada

This book is dedicated with love to my three sons,

Connor,

Jude,

and Lochlan.

My life is incredible because you boys are in it.

Acknowledgements

I would like to first thank my partner, Marni McCarthy, who, without her love and support, the dream of writing this book would have never been realized. Also for never being afraid to voice her opinion, and whose brilliance and critical thinking skills are unmatched. I would also like to thank Jack McCarthy for conducting an emergency, last second edit and Marion and Minirva and the rest of the McCarthy's for allowing me to borrow their daughter, sister, and mother.

Integral to the completion of this project was Mishell Raedeke of Graphic Design Concepts who is an artistic genius and Jill Veitch of Webb Publishing for formatting under intense time constraints. Also, Ryan and Jenn Grundy of Atomic 55 Internet Technologies and David Miles of Montgomery Miles law firm.

I would like to thank all my teachers, co-workers, and clients, who I have learned so much from through the years, especially Michelle Colter, Tom Schooley, and Giovanni Vidotto who have been great supports and have had incredible patience in engaging me in healthy debate.

Finally, I would like to thank my family. My mother, Arlene Elliott who, in addition to writing her own book, has done more work than anyone over the last two years to help make my project a reality. I would also like to express gratitude to my father, Michael Douglas, who taught us to never let go of our dreams, and to my brother, Aaron Douglas, for his support and encouragement; you'll always be the Chief to me.

Contents

Introduction

This book will NOT change your life. Nor will any other book, news article, counseling session, diet, or late-night television program. Only *you* have the power to change your life. The next hundred-plus pages are devoted to teaching you how to maximize your potential and harness your power by understanding the connection between your biological, psychological, and environmental systems. This is a human operator's manual that will serve as a guide to teach you ways of optimizing your functioning psychologically, physiologically, and emotionally. By reading this book you will have clear instructions on how to operate yourself-something that we all so desperately need. This will enable you to better understand human functioning and take control of how you are operating yourself.

I am a counselor, not a scientist. What you are about to read is a culmination of my studies and professional practice. In my initial years of counseling, I found myself grasping for tools outside of what my formal education of counseling and psychology had to offer. I began to study the fields of biology, physiology, and mind-body medicine with the goal of creating a treatment for my clients that would help them not only identify problems and symptoms, but also move beyond them by harnessing their own power and maximizing their potential to create health and wellness. This book is born from years of study and practice. It is an understandable operation's manual to help individuals take control of their functioning and choose how to operate themselves. This reminds me of a story.

My dad has an old VCR that he totes with him every time he

moves. For those of you who don't remember what a VCR is, it's like a large old-fashioned DVD player that you insert giant tapes into so that you can watch movies. There is a whole generation of baby boomers living today who, like my father, have yet to figure out how to set the digital clock on their VCR, let alone how to program it to record. Many are unsure how to connect it to their television. They are enslaved to the dark ages of technology, and reliant on the goodwill of friends and relatives to help them set up their system. For this task, my father relies on me.

Not only am I kind enough to hook the VCR up to the TV, but I even set the clock and leave him an easy-to-read chart outlining the conversion rate from the twenty-four-hour clock to the twelve-hour system.

As soon as I finish, the first thing he does is test to see if I installed the VCR correctly by loading a giant videocassette tape, picking up the remote, and pressing *play*. Pressing *play* is never as easy as it sounds. Even though he has had the same remote for over twenty years, he is committed to inputting the correct information. He reads every button on the remote before finally settling on the function that he desires; then applies the appropriate amount of pressure to the button. He holds the remote in one hand and depresses the button with the other, causing the red light to blink, which indicates that the transaction is in process. Two hours later, I usually receive several phone calls questioning me on how to change the input on the VCR to cable so that he can watch a regular television program. The point of this story is that without the instruction manual or someone with the required knowledge to guide him, my dad's technology is useless. This principle can also be applied to humans.

Humans were given the most complex and efficient machine on the planet but were never taught how to operate it properly. Even if they had been given detailed instructions, most would have chosen not to read them, since the machine operates reasonably well without them. This is true for my dad's old VCR, but to get the most out of his machine, he needs to read the manual. Not having the instruction manual is fine if you want to get by with the basics, but if you want a bigger, better, happier life, you must pick up those instructions, read them carefully, and take control of your functioning.

If you were an expert sailor and had decided to sail to Hawaii, the first thing you would do would be to get a compass and a nautical map so that you could plot your course. You wouldn't just hop into your boat, pull up anchor, and hope that the currents would get you to your destination. Most people approach life this way and find themselves in situations that they never would have consciously chosen to be in. They hopped aboard, pulled up anchor, and set sail letting the current of life direct their path, rather than choosing a course of action to give them the desired results. Often, this passive approach lands them in my office or in the offices of my colleagues. Simply reacting to the world without ever consciously choosing what you want is a recipe for an unhappy, unfulfilled life. I used to be guilty of this myself, but not anymore. My life is too important to float around and deal with whatever life may bring me and I believe that yours is too.

This operator's manual will not only help you take control of how you manage yourself, but will challenge you to provide yourself with clear, concise direction. You may have to navigate around some obstacles to get where you want to go, but you are capable. You can set a course of action, stay on track, and move in the direction that you want your life to be going.

The foundation of the process is *taking control* of how you operate yourself physically, emotionally, and psychologically. Evolution has brought us to a point where we can make conscious choices, and it is now up to us to maximize our functioning and live fulfilling lives. Otherwise, what's the point?

The human system has developed over thousands of years. Complex biological survival mechanisms have evolved over time, enabling our species to thrive no matter what challenge we faced. Modern science has been able to identify these mechanisms and determine how they operate. However, we were never given an instruction manual, and because our culture has changed so much over the past one hundred years, out-evolving our genes, which take thousands of years to adapt, we find ourselves having many complex problems.

As we sit in our office chairs staring blankly at the computer screen, these same survival mechanisms are actually working against us. Some of their by-products are anxiety, stress, weight gain, fatigue, irrational fears, and procrastination. This manual will teach you how to take control of these survival mechanisms and control how they are functioning.

I work predominantly in the field of addictions and this is especially true in this industry. After observing countless people successfully quit using drugs and alcohol only to return to active use within a short period of time, I committed myself to creating better results. With this dedication, I studied, researched, and experimented (no, not *that* way) in order to enhance my technique and skill level with the hope that I could help my clients achieve better results. The problem that I found with the addictions field is that the foundational principles conflict with modern, cutting-edge science. The addictions field evolved in a time period when people believed that the brain was fixed at age 18 and remained that way for life. Today, we know that this is simply not true. The human brain changes throughout the lifespan and we can consciously choose to guide its development. With this knowledge, combined with understanding how the body operates, and how to control their physical functioning, clients learned to better manage themselves, and stick to their goals even through intense physiological craving states. This has resulted in helping people make massive changes in their lives. I have found that by teaching people this concept whom struggle with other issues, such as anxiety and depression, also benefit with incredible results. People are able to take better control of their functioning, reduce their physical symptoms, and live healthier and happier lives.

After watching people make remarkable, sustained changes in their lives, I decided to write this book and make this information accessible to everyone so that they too could have the knowledge and skills necessary to take control of how they operate themselves. Taking conscious control of your functioning radically changes how you live your life.

This book provides the tools required to control your functioning and teaches you how to create an operator's manual specific to you. Not only will you learn how to break old habits, you will also find insight into why the habits developed in the first place. You will learn how to 'install' new healthy habits that will move you in the direction you want to go in life.

There are many experts who offer general guidelines on how the human body operates. These principles will not relate exactly the same for each individual reader so it is up to you to take these principles and fold them into your own functioning. You must remain critical and thoughtful. If something in this book isn't working for you and you have tried alternative ways to express it into your life, then simply dismiss it and move on. You are the expert on your life, and *only you* have the power to take control and maximize your own functioning.

Consciously operating yourself will provide you with increased control over your life, allowing you to experience enhanced relationships, and live a happier, healthier life. Only you have the power to choose to read this book and take control of how you operate yourself. It's time to pick up the remote of your life and take control of how you operate yourself.

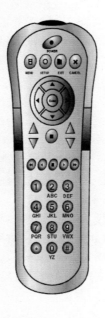

Chapter 1

Operating Yourself for Optimal Performance

"Knowledge is power and consequently, knowledge
of self provides self-empowerment."
Bruce Lipton, *Biology of Belief* (2005)

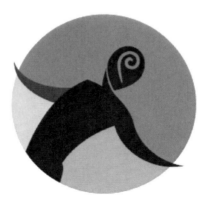

Imagine in this instant, your past was wiped away and any insecurity you've ever had was gone. What if that little voice in your head that undermines you and keeps you from thriving was torn away from you and you were left with nothing but strength and hope? How would your life change?

How would your life change if by simply understanding the purpose to your fears and insecurities allowed you to be liberated from them? What if they provided you with a specific biological survival function and by making a few simple changes could allow you to silence that voice in your head and with it all your fears and insecurities?

I want to offer you a new way of functioning. I want to give you the power of control. I want to give you control of your life, control of your body, control of your thoughts, fears, anxieties, and emotions. I want to give you the power to take charge of your emotions rather than being led around by them. You are in control and are about to learn how to take this control. You are about to receive the power necessary to take control of your functioning and learn how to operate yourself for optimal performance. The choice is yours. You can take your lead from that little voice in your head that undermines what you are striving to be or do, or you can take control of that voice and empower yourself to be in charge.

Many people move through life reacting to what the outside world presents to them. When they are wronged, they blame. When they are rewarded, they smile and relax. When it rains, they huddle inside and when it's sunny, they head to the beach. They wear a shirt that feels good until someone disapproves. Then they hide it in the back of their closet, replacing it with one they are told looks better. Most people are controlled by doing what they are told, while others are controlled by doing the opposite of what they are told. Few people take the time to consciously decide for themselves what they want and what feels right to them, rarely putting in the effort to decide what state they want to approach life in and how they want to operate themselves. You are in control of your mood, feelings, thoughts, and actions. Few people take this opportunity to take control of how they operate themselves. This book will break down your biological mechanisms and teach you how to take control of your functioning to operate yourself for maximum effectiveness. The choice is yours. Let me tell you what led to the construction of this book.

My Journey

After graduating with an undergraduate degree in psychology, I had a life-changing epiphany: I was qualified to be a damn fine waiter, but not much else! So I pressed on and obtained a master's degree in counseling and found employment working in the field of mental health and addictions. It was there that I came to a second life-changing epiphany: the field of counseling can be dangerous and a lot of well-meaning counselors are actually creating more problems than they are helping to solve.

I went into the "helping profession" to do exactly that—help people. I wanted to make a positive difference in people's lives and maybe even effect a little change in the world. There is no taste quite as pure as when innocence meets naivety. Well, it didn't take too long for me to realize that the skills and techniques I had learned in university were helping people feel better about their situations, but not actually helping them make any real changes. This assertion resonated with some of my colleagues.

I came to realize that most people don't actually want to make any real life changes due to discomfort, fear, and a strong aversion to hard work. People wanted to feel better about their lives without actually making any changes. They wanted to feel better about living in a thorn bush without actually doing anything to get out of the thorns. My job was to help them reframe the thorn bush, renaming it a rose bush. Then they could feel better about their situation and thank their kind hearted counselor, who did such an amazing job in not actually helping them with anything, because their situation was still the same. People can be quite appreciative when you help them make this reframe.

Unfortunately for me, this approach wasn't good enough. I realized that I was actively participating in the continuation of the problem. The bar I held for myself was higher; I wanted to help people get out of the thorns altogether. Some of my colleagues were on the same page that I was, while others were happy with the thankfulness that they received from their clients. Others maintain such a professional disconnect from their clients that keeps them safely away from their successes or repeated failures, and also prevents them from examining their paradigm of therapy. I do agree that you can't take on your client's failures, but if you are helping them to reframe the thorn bush, in my opinion, you are part of the problem and just another thorn keeping people stuck in their place. This is how counselors sometimes contribute to the problem. The following story is a prime example of this.

One day a woman walked into my office. She was on top of the world, she was absolutely beaming. She told me that she had just returned from "treatment" and that she was ecstatic. For those who don't know what "treatment" in the addictions field means, it refers to a residential treatment program where people struggling with alcohol or drug dependencies go to "get fixed." Unfortunately, the success statistics on this billion-dollar industry are minimal at best. Residential treatment centers traditionally don't maintain thorough research methods to collect statistics that measure their effectiveness. However, the statistics that are available routinely report that one year after treatment less than approximately 18 percent of people who completed the program, remain abstinent from drug and/or alcohol use. Residential treatment is seen as the "magic bullet," the cure-all of the addictions industry, and like most cure-alls, it is ineffective and may even be damaging to client's success as it often sets people up for failure.

For this woman, like most leaving a treatment center, she was beaming and ready to take on the world. From my desire to be the best counselor I could be, I asked her what happened at treatment that provided her with such a profound change. She replied that she had "finally, after all these years, dealt with her past issues." If I had a nickel for every time I have heard that phrase...

I saw her for a few sessions, and like a lot of people who are doing well, she stopped attending therapy, and rightly so, as she no longer needed counseling. Six months passed and she was back in my office. Her life was in shambles and she was breaking down into tears. She was using crack cocaine daily again, and asserted that she needed "to go back to treatment." I asked her why she wanted to return to treatment, and she replied, "I need to deal with my past issues."

Stunned, I replied, "last time you were here and feeling on top of the world, you stated that you finally, after all these years, had dealt with your past issues."

She replied, "Yes, but now they are back."

This is a prime example of the potential danger of counseling. As counselors, we are taught to examine and re-examine a person's past until they gain insight, and that this insight will result in change. This is a myth that the field of psychology has innocently perpetuated for years. The truth is that insight alone won't create change-people need to take action to create change. All the good in psychology has been discounted by the pervasive repetition of the belief that all problems stem from Freud's theories of childhood development and trauma.

As I studied how the human brain operates, I realized that what we were doing in therapy was counter-productive. What the field of neuroscience, the study of the brain, has unveiled in the last five years calls into question the past hundred years of therapeutic dogma. We don't need to perpetually deal with the past every time we make a mistake or feel some painful feelings. Pain is an indicator that something is wrong in the present and that we need to pay attention. It is our guide that tells us that things aren't perfect and it is time to make change.

The idea that your subconscious is a black box that fills up with trauma, and only through banging away at the past with your friendly neighborhood psychoanalytic therapist can you empty the box, is scientifically dated. Freud, the well-dressed, pipe-smoking, beard-wearing, cocaine-pushing, "founding father" of psychology, was wrong. I repeat-Freud's premise was faulty. Freud believed that through psychoanalysis people take their metaphorical bucket of symptoms that was filled up through traumatic experience, out into the backyard and dump it into the trash, thus removing any negative emotional or psychological symptom. Unfortunately, the bucket gets filled back up through life experience and then you have to start the process all over again, beginning with your birth. I don't want to discount the important contributions that Freud made to the field of psychology, but as a field, we held on to the wrong message and for far too long. This created a past-, symptom-focused field that is reactive to problems instead of teaching people how to maximize their functioning, or focusing on what people are doing well, and building on that success.

I am committed to helping people get out of the thorn bush and move beyond the past, which is why I created this operator's manual. I wanted to counter these problems and give people something that they could use without fear and discomfort, that wouldn't require so much work that people would rather do nothing. I wanted it to be science-based, proactive, and solution-focused that gives people easy to use solutions to move them towards happiness and health rather than just a mere absence of symptoms. This book cuts through all the dogma, faulty beliefs, and assumptions to enable people to create true, lasting change.

Chris Douglas

Chapter 2

Human Development

"Man's mind, once stretched by a new idea,
never regains its original dimension."

Oliver Wendell Holmes, Jr.

The Briefcase

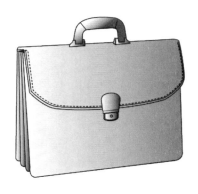

Michael was born on November 8, 1951. He was one of seven children and dreamed of playing hockey in the NHL. Money was tight, as his father was a factory worker at the Ford Motor plant in Ontario. Living in a two bedroom apartment above a beauty salon in a poverty stricken area of Mississauga, his family struggled. Michael struggled too. He attended a Catholic school in the heart of Mississauga where, from the beginning, he struggled with kindergarten but was moved on to grade one, where his difficulties would continue. At the end of the first grade he was held back, repeating the grade once then moving forward the next year, mostly due to his age. He failed grade two, but was advanced due to his age. In grade three he failed again, this time repeating the grade. At the end of his second try he was advanced, again mostly due to his age. Despite struggling in grade four, five and six he continued to be moved forward mostly due to his age. At the end of grade six his teacher Mrs. Lawless called Michael's parents into the office. His father had to work so only his mother could attend. Mrs. Lawless recommended that Michael be put into a special school for children with developmental disabilities. Michael was horrified as his friends labeled this school the "funny farm."

All through school, Michael excelled in sports. He had many friends and was well liked; he compensated for his difficulties by being the class clown. But, this was all about to change.

If he stayed in Catholic school he would be held back. If he went to the "funny farm" he would be ridiculed. The teacher explained to Michael's mother how at this alternative school Michael would excel as he would learn "special skills" such as how to stock a grocery store shelf. Michael's mother knew he was capable of more and somewhere locked deep inside of himself, Michael knew this too.

This decision weighed heavily on his mother as she knew she had to find a better way. Alone and desperate for help she took Michael to Dr. Murphy, a pediatrician. Upon hearing the situation, Dr. Murphy admitted Michael to the Toronto Hospital for Sick Children where he stayed for a full week. The assessment results indicated that there were no developmental disabilities nor was there anything physically wrong with Michael, which would prevent him from being successful in school. Dr. Murphy suggested that there may be something psychological going on with him, some sort of block preventing him from thriving. Today he would have had the opportunity to sample twenty different kinds of medication, but this was not the case in the early 1960's.

Upon hearing this news Michael's mother decided to try another option and pulled Michael out of Catholic school, registering him in public school. Michael was a hard worker and being from a large family with a low income he learned to save his money. He saved every penny he earned from his paper route and kept it hidden from his two little brothers whom he shared a bedroom with.

For Michael it was the summer after grade six, and knowing that he was going to public school in September, he knew he had to make a change. Instead of spending the summer playing baseball and hockey in the streets with his friends, he took his money down to the general store where he bought himself a big, brown, leather briefcase. To him briefcases represented success and intelligence: his teachers all carried briefcases with them at school, and he would see successful looking business men carrying them around in their expensive suits.

He knew he had to reinvent himself, and to him getting a new briefcase meant success. Michael wanted success in school more than anything. He was done being the "dumb kid," the "class clown," and the "jock." He desperately wanted to be the smart kid and at the tender age of twelve made this transformation the only way he could imagine: by buying a briefcase.

Knowing that good readers went to the library, he stormed down there and started to check books out. He reasoned that the bigger and heavier the book, the smarter the person would have to be to read it. So Michael found the heaviest books he could find, and although they were way above his reading comprehension, he stuffed these books into his briefcase until he could barely close it. He was a great athlete, but his arms weren't prepared for the weight of these books in his briefcase and he struggled to carry them home.

Michael spent all hours of the day carrying his briefcase full of books up and down the street in a trancelike state. At first he was crying for being so "dumb," and then started to tell himself "I am smart." In time the tears subsided as did the hurt, failure, and feeling of being "dumb." Slowly, he started believing that he was smart. Michael let go of his dream of becoming a hockey player and instead pictured himself as a teacher standing in front of a classroom instructing students. As the mileage accumulated, the hurt dissipated, paving way for the new Michael. He envisioned himself as a "nerd." He was no longer the class clown, the jock, he was smart.

A short while into summer he met another "nerd." Someone he wouldn't have even noticed a few months back, but the timing was right. Like attracts like, and nerd attracted nerd. When Michael wasn't walking the streets to and from the library repeating his "I am smart" mantra, he was at his friend's house reading comic books. With his new belief that he was smart and the time spent reading comic books, his reading skills caught up enough that for the first time in his young life Michael legitimately passed grade seven. He then passed grades eight and nine and continued on until he eventually got a Bachelor and a Master's degree in Social Work. He moved on to become a professor at a college and fulfilled his vision of becoming a teacher. Michael specialized in teaching students how to work with people with developmental disabilities.

A few years later he was back in Ontario visiting his mother and she asked him, "Michael do you remember that big brown briefcase you bought in grade six." As if struck by lightening he flashed back to the moment when he changed the course of his life. His path then became clear as he made the connection from his past experiences to his present life. His early experiences served as an important teaching ground to give him a sense of purpose to help others who were struggling, failing and feeling the shame that accompanied them. Michael went on to have two sons: one became a successful actor, and the other, an author of a book written to help people take control of how they operate themselves.

This is an amazing, true story of how a child completely changed how he was operating himself. We all have this power inside. If a child can make this incredible transformation, than anyone can. The turning point of Michael's transition towards success was in acquiring the briefcase, his symbol of change and success.

The Three Brains

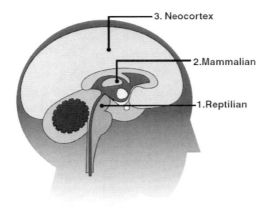

In biology, evolution is the process from which traits are passed down from generation to generation. Every organism alive today, including plants and animals is a product of evolution dating back to when the earth first formed 4.5 billion years ago. Reptiles emerged 300 million years ago, preceding mammals which evolved 200 million years ago. Finally, humans evolved approximately 200 thousand years ago. This evolutionary trend is emulated within human development. Within our human brain, we can trace our evolution into three distinct categories of structures that are layered one on top of the other. At the base is the brain stem which is also known as the reptilian brain. On top of this structure is the limbic system also known as the mammalian brain. The top part of the brain is what makes us human and is known as the neocortex, which means new brain. The three brains are complex and interconnected with each other, but only the neocortex is aware of the existence of the other two. The neocortex is the control panel of human functioning and directs the other two brains with conscious intent. Without conscious intent the mammalian brain often takes over and many people find themselves operating from this level, resulting in the emergence of many difficulties.

These three brains-the reptilian, mammalian, and neocortex are interconnected, yet responsible for separate tasks. They developed in order of 'survival need.' First, the reptilian emerged to keep us safe from external threats; then came the mammalian brain to protect us from internal threats; finally, the neocortex developed to give us advanced community, cooperation, and intelligence as we aren't physically as strong as most members of the reptile and mammal community. Difficulties often arise as each level isn't consciously aware of the level above it, however the higher the layer the more control.

The instinctual reptilian brain reacts to directions from the mammalian brain as a survival reflex, but it doesn't have the ability for conscious understanding of the existence of the mammalian. The mammalian brain takes direction from the neocortex but isn't aware of its existence as there is no consciousness or logic at this level of functioning. The mammalian brain cannot differentiate between information collected by our senses from thoughts from the neocortex. Therefore, it cannot distinguish reality perceived through our senses from thoughts from the neocortex. In other words it cannot differentiate thoughts ("synthetic reality") from perceived reality ("real reality").

The reptilian brain operates at the most basic level of survival. It includes the functions of respiration, digestion, circulation, and reproduction. This is the most primitive and instinctual part of our brain.

The main function of the mammalian brain is to operate our basic emotions, memory, and motivation. This is where emotion and physical sensations are attached to memory. At this level emotions are simply the chemical communication signals that get converted into physical sensations, which our conscious mind identifies as emotions. The mammalian brain also houses our reward and fear pathways giving us pleasure and pain, which are essential to motivation. It is located directly on top of the reptilian brain and builds on that level of functioning.

The neocortex is the pinnacle of evolution. This is what makes us human and translates into "neo" meaning "new" and "cortex" meaning "brain," thus new brain. This final part to develop gives us the control panel for our functioning. This is the reason we have language, creativity, abstract thought, logic, and the ability to make conscious decisions. All our executive functions such as goal-setting, cost-benefit analysis, anticipating events, planning, empathy and decision-making are housed in this part of the brain. It is the CEO of human operations and is what differentiates us from animals and other mammals, as we have proportionally much bigger cortexes.

These parts and their functions are repeated several times throughout this book as repetition enhances understanding. By the time you are done reading, you will have a simple, working knowledge base of how these parts function and what they mean to your ability to control how you operate yourself.

Later on I will discuss how different parts operate and how they change or stop the functioning of one another. This is an oversimplification for understanding purposes because no part of the human body ever stops working-otherwise, you would likely be headed for surgery or already dead. If a part stopped working completely it would harden and die off.

As always, consult a physician before trying a new routine or diet and exercise program, and in addition, consult yourself. You are the pilot of your life. You are the one who reaps the rewards or pays the consequences of your choices. You only get one shot at life, so make sure you are living yours and not someone else's. If something doesn't make sense on a logical level then get more information. If someone's advice or something in this book doesn't ring true to you then listen to yourself. If something doesn't seem right to you at the gut level, it probably won't work for you. Get more information, try something else, but most importantly listen to the encouraging voice in your head. This voice is coming from the neocortex.

Don't limit yourself. What one human is capable of, we are all capable of. We may not be able to run the 100m in 9.69 seconds like Usain Bolt, but we are all capable of running. We may not be able to amass a multi-billion-dollar fortune like Bill Gates, but we can take control of our finances and become wealthy. Letting go of the limits that hold you in place and allowing yourself to start running, or begin investing, you never know what may happen. I am always amazed how quickly things start to fall into place when people start to work for themselves and build some positive momentum, how dramatically their life changes for the better. This power is within all of us. You never know-you may find yourself breaking a world record or building a fortune-five-hundred company. When you start to let go of the self-imposed limitations that hold you in place, you will astonish yourself as you discover what you are truly capable of.

Finally, there is a popular misconception around change. Well-meaning counselors like myself at one point, will tell you that change is a process, that it takes time, and is very difficult. Change isn't a process, nor is it an option. People are always changing, developing, and growing. Change only stops when we are dead. We can fight change and draw it out, or we can embrace it and make some conscious choices to take action, which inevitably speeds things up. Or we can lie around, fight it, and end up with change being forced upon us, which research has shown to decrease human performance. Take a leap, move forward and direct your life. Change isn't a process; retraining may be a process, but it's one that we can facilitate with movement. If you want to quit drinking, lose weight, or live healthier, you have to take action, or else retraining will come slow. As for change, it is unavoidable.

Our human system has developed for survival and efficiency. This is what allowed our species to survive for the last two hundred thousand years while other species have vanished. Understanding the three levels of the brain and corresponding physical attributes is a necessary foundation in taking control of your functioning.

Chris Douglas

Chapter 3

The Reptilian Brain

"The man who never alters his opinions is like standing water,
and breeds reptiles of the mind."

William Blake

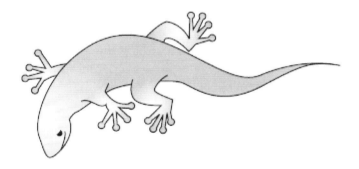

Paralyzed in Fear

Amanda was a loving, stay at home mom of three children who
were now in their teen years and not in need of as much day to day
care. Her husband worked out of town and was away for months at
a time. At home she excelled, the house was spotless, and the kids
had their lunches packed and homework done every day. When it
came to leaving the house she was like a frightened child scared to

walk into the dark. She was debilitated. She fit the diagnostic criteria for agoraphobia, but her problem went much deeper than that. Even the thought of having to go to the grocery store caused her to have a panic attack. She felt out of control, helpless. She knew she needed help long ago but was so afraid to leave the house she waited until her pain was so intense that she knew she had no other choice, but to go for help. When she finally arrived at my office for help, it was her husband who brought her there, and did most of the talking. He explained his perception of the problem and made it clear that if things did not change he was going to leave her. He stated that they had not had an evening out of the house for almost fifteen years. He loved her, but her world had become so small there was no room for him in it. The entire first session focused on creating a plan on how she could attend the next session without becoming too anxious to leave the house.

I could tell what was happening, her reptilian brain had gone haywire and every time she had a remote thought of change, she had panic attacks and her fear response would kick in with so much intensity she was paralyzed in fear.

The purpose of the reptilian brain is safety and it operates from instinct. Its main functions of respiration, digestion, circulation and reproduction are essential to survival. The reptilian brain operates the muscles and skeletal system which gives us form, structure, strength and most important of all, mobility. It is designed to help us survive the harsh outside world and gives us the strength and speed needed to accomplish this task. Consider the age of the dinosaur. Dinosaurs were the mightiest reptiles of all. They were primarily operated from instinct, instinct to survive. There was no higher brain functioning and consequently they did not create contingency plans to deal with such inevitabilities as a meteor striking the earth, or an ice age. For Amanda, her survival instinct flared up every time she had a thought of leaving the house.

She first needed to learn the skills necessary to calm her inner reptile.

When your survival mechanisms fire up a combination of physiological responses occur. Your breathing becomes shallow as your lungs attempt to flood your muscles with oxygen necessary to run short sprints to get away from danger, or to make you strong enough to fight off an enemy. Your lungs take in less air, but push it out to the rest of your body at a much higher rate. However this is also what leads some people to have panic attacks as they hyperventilate and start to think that they are going to die. Your heart rate and blood pressure increase to aid in getting the oxygen to the muscles, essential organs and the reptilian brain in order to support the increase of speed, strength and instinctual decision making. The stress hormones of adrenaline and cortisol are also released to maximize strength and speed. Blood flow to the top part of the brain and stomach is decreased as it is rerouted to the survival mechanisms. You don't want to waste energy digesting a steak or over thinking what to do when a tiger is chasing you. For Amanda, her first line of defense was to learn to breathe properly. She needed to learn to elongate her breathing in order to slow her heart rate and turn off her survival mechanisms.

The instinctual reptilian brain works much like the dinosaur brain as it reads and reacts to the surrounding environment, with no time to slow things down for complex thought. It simply replies to environmental stimuli quickly and helps us survive external threats. It evolved to survive harsh environments. It is designed to move, not sit in an office chair, or on a couch. When trained, the human reptile is capable of magnificent feats. Remember the example of Usain Bolt who ran 100 meters in 9.69 seconds. It is the reptilian part that makes this possible.

The human reptile's strength is its adaptability. With instinct, there is no emotion, thought or intelligence. This is why reptiles make bad pets, they will never know their name, or come when you call them, and they are incapable of love.

The human reptile is responsible for the survival mechanisms and includes the stress hormones. Like Amanda, spending too much time with the survival system turned on your system starts to break down and as you tune your survival system to the world around you it gets easier and easier to switch into survival mode. This reveals itself in intense anxious states.

Energy Systems

We have two basic energy systems that we operate from. We have a calming system and an activating system. The calming system is called the parasympathetic nervous system (PSNS) and the activating system is known as the sympathetic nervous system (SNS). When we are in the calming system our body can grow and repair itself. When we are in the activating system our body is revving up getting ready to move, and if need be go into fight, flight or freeze mode.

Fight is when we attack an external threat like if you see a coyote attacking your child and you beat it off with a tennis racket. This is an automatic response that your body undergoes without the need for complex thought. In flight, we run from danger like if you are camping and you see a bear turn towards you from a hundred feet away. Your body will switch into the activating mode and run yourself to safety before questioning whether or not the bear was going to chase you. Finally in freeze mode, you are close to the bear so your body tenses up, frozen and unable to move with the hope that the bear senses no threat from you or doesn't see you there. Or if you are stepping off a curb and see a bus about to hit you and despite not being in a balanced position you freeze up long enough for the bus to pass without hitting you. Then you finish your step forward. For Amanda, she became frozen with fear, giving her the feeling that she was paralyzed. As she learned how to manage her fear response at the reptilian level she slowly regained a sense of control over her anxiety.

We can manage what energy system we are in by deep breathing. This will be discussed more in depth later, but is important in operating your reptilian brain and survival system. We process food differently depending on which energy state we are in when we eat the food. When you are in the calming system food gets fully processed, extracting all the nutrients. In the activating system your body's focus is on movement and the blood that would normally be sent to your stomach is routed to your muscles for movement. This basically shuts down digestion and decreases the proper processing of food and nutrients that happens when you are in the calming system. Taking between five and ten deep diaphragmatic breathes switches you from the activating SNS response into the calming PSNS state.

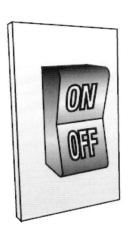

State Management

The second way to switch your arousal state and take control of you survival response is through state management. Tears of joy have a different chemical composition then tears of sadness. The same holds true for your physical state. Picture someone who is depressed. Typically their head will be lowered, facing the ground, shoulders slumped and they will look physically withdrawn. Now picture someone who is confident and happy. Typically they will have their head up, shoulders back, be smiling and appear open and connected with the world. There is a different chemical composition for each of these states. Often when we are in an emotional state we can change it by simply changing our body posture which releases a different combination of chemicals within the body.

For Amanda starting with deep breathing to calm her fear response and managing her physical state allowed her to take control of some of her anxious symptoms. This was the start she needed to build on in learning to take control of how she was operating herself. At first she was constantly deep breathing throughout the day to stay in the calming system, but as time passed and her breathing skills enhanced, she needed to monitor her breathing less, and less.

Capabilities of the Human Reptile

The human reptile can be tamed and ultimately controlled by your higher brain functions. However, as it requires no thought to operate it, it is an automatic process to help you survive. Like a fine surgical instrument it can be sharpened to enhance its functioning.

Often most people do not take conscious control of its development, or work to get it into peak shape. What is your human reptile capable of? Is it in peak physical health?

In India there was a young boy named Budhia Singh. I use this story to illustrate a point and do not want to open the debate whether this was child abuse or not as I don't know all the factors. Budhia has ran up to 60 kilometers on several occasions, but found himself in the Limca Book of Records in 2006 at age four, for running an astonishing 7 hour 65 kilometer marathon without water. This raises the question, what are the rest of us capable of?

Again, take the amazing feats of Usain Bolt running 100 meters in 9.69 seconds, or the 200 meters in 19.30, or with his teammates breaking the world and Olympic records by running the 4X100 meter relay in 37.10 seconds. What more are you capable of? Javier Sotomayor of Cuba broke the world record by high jumping an incredible eight feet in the air. Or take Mike Powell, of the U.S. who long jumped 8.95 meters. We are all capable of more and what one human can do we are all capable of to some degree. Maybe you don't want to sharpen your Olympic skills, but we are all capable of more. Even these amazing athletes who may be as close to peak physical shape as possible have room to grow and develop themselves in one way or another.

So how do you operate yourself physically? Are you consciously in control, or do you eat and exercise in reaction to your emotional state or from a reptilian place of instinct rather than higher thought? There are two ways we can dramatically alter our physical shape. No surprise that this is through diet and exercise. However, this is not about following some expert's advice that appeared on some paid late night television ad, arguing that if you only follow their program you will lose 63 pounds in four and a half days. This is about observing for yourself how you are functioning after your body processes food and how that is related to your activity level. The "experts" can be helpful, but you must listen to the most important expert of them all, your body. Paying attention to how your body reacts to something either positive or negative will reconnect you to the intuition of your body and clearly demonstrate how you need to fuel yourself and move to optimize your physical functioning. Of course, getting some help or following someone else's routine may increase your rate of success, but you need to be mindful to the body's indicators that tell if what you are doing is working or not.

This is about communication. We communicate with our body in two ways. Through what we feed it and how we move it. Reptiles, animals, and mammals have natural biorhythms as do humans. However, we tend to be the only species that is so disconnected from our natural environment and biorhythms. I don't see a lot of bears reading about outdoor life in the newspaper in front of their air conditioner, yet I can give you a long list of humans that do.

Brown bear's mate in springtime, fatten themselves up in fall and find a cave to hibernate in during winter when they have their babies, sometimes without even waking up. The baby bears nurse until springtime when they learn to find food. Between age two and three they will be sent away to design their own life. Female bears are ready to mate between four and seven years old and the cycle starts over again. This cycle has been followed since brown bears evolved.

Humans used to have clearer life patterns based on their food source and location in the world. Today our society is safe and riddled with grocery stores and restaurants. We no longer need to follow the biorhythms of our food as we have food from all over the world available to us at any given moment. Today we dictate our diet, instead of relying on the available food source based on location and time of year. This has enabled us to hibernate in our houses, and eat whatever we want at any time of the year, disconnecting us from our natural patterns. This has resulted in incongruence between our culture and genetics, as our society has undergone drastic change within the last hundred years, while it takes thousand of years for our genes to evolve.

Communicating with the Human Reptile

We communicate with our body through movement and food which becomes a reflection of our lifestyle. It is our lifestyle that creates the reflection that we see in the mirror. If we change the way we communicate with our body, our reflection changes. You can change the message you are communicating through changing your fuel source and/or changing your movement. Do you communicate that you are getting ready to hibernate by sitting on the couch all day, growing deposits of fat to keep you comfortable and warm? Or do you communicate that you are Usain Bolt and ready to sprint into life at any given moment? What message are you sending your body? Are you telling it to slow your metabolism by feeding it high calorie, low nutrition food? Or are you sending the message that you are human and alive by eating natural organic, unprocessed food like an apple or banana? Are you communicating that your lifestyle requires movement, agility and speed, or docility and minimal energy? What message are you sending?

Remember those sandwich commercials starring a 425 pound man named Jared? Jared's miraculous change was not about the sandwich! Sure he changed his primary fuel source, but he also changed the message he was communicating to his body. The first sequence of commercials had people noting that Jared was up and walking. Later he introduced us to his favorite "low fat" sandwiches. Jared eventually went from 425 pounds down to 190.

He did this by changing the message he sent to his body. He no longer communicated docility and a state of hibernation through a high fat low nutritional yield diet. He communicated movement and supplied food that energized his body instead of taking energy away from it making him tired, ready to nap, or lie in bed watching television. When the reptilian brain understood the message that hibernation was over and Jared's lifestyle required more agility, and movement, his body responded by becoming lighter, leaner, and quicker. Unlike most other dieters, Jared continued to send this message to his body and maintained his improved shape instead of reverting to his previous pattern of living.

Food as Fuel

The most influential method of communication with our body is through food. It is not just about what we eat, but also how we eat, why we are eating and the timing of when we eat. Sumo wrestlers who are trying to put on weight for a competition do not actually increase the calories that they are eating, but change the timing of when they eat. Instead of spreading their calories throughout the day they get up during the night and pack their calorie load in around sleep times. This process keeps their body from burning the calories as they get stored as fat on to their frame. How do you feel after a big meal where you over eat? Are you tired? How about after eating an apple or some fruit? Are you tired, or do you feel energized and ready for action? This is not about giving you a list of what to eat or not to eat, this is about discovering what food energizes you for your self. Only you can make this determination.

I ran into one woman who attended a talk I gave where I

discussed this process of changing the message you are communicating to the body and she told me that she had lost thirty pounds by tuning into her body this way. She stated that she started to focus on how she wanted to feel thirty minutes after she ate instead of focusing on what would satisfy her cravings in the moment and ate accordingly. She created a list of foods that put her in the state she wanted to be in and worked on adding those to her diet, instead of focusing on what she couldn't have. This was enough to disrupt her pattern of eating based on what she felt like in the moment and limited emotional eating. This is a small change that only affects the psychology around eating, but she identified that it worked better than any diet or exercise program she had ever tried. As it was based on what works for her body, and was directed by her rather than someone who doesn't know how her body operates on an individual level. This is about finding what works for you, so experiment and listen to your body.

It is important to make a connection between the symptoms of your body running poorly versus operating yourself with maximum efficiency. Typically feeling lethargic, bloated or exhausted are the signs of poor functioning, while feeling lean, alive and filled with vitality are often indicative of operating at a higher level. The next two exercises are designed to bring you closer to your desired state.

Make a food list of what you have eaten in the last few days. Write it down and note how you felt approximately thirty minutes after you have eaten. If you cannot remember what you have eaten or how you have felt start by experimenting with what you eat and spend a week monitoring how you feel afterwards. I'm sure on a logical level you can narrow down this list, but try to have some fun with this.

Here is a random list:

> French fries
>
> Potato Chips
>
> Almonds
>
> Chicken
>
> Coffee
>
> Water
>
> Cucumber
>
> Ice cream
>
> Apples
>
> Turkey sandwich

Become your own nutritional expert. Your body will tell you by how it functions what is good for it or not. In the 1970's the experts argued for low carbohydrate, high protein, high fat eating. In the 1980's they said we should eat three meals a day, no snacks and should be counting calories as "all calories are created equal." In the 1990's we were told avoid fat at all costs, and health equaled eating low fat. Then at the turn of the millennium we were told to go back to low carbohydrate, high protein, and to eat many small meals a day to keep our metabolism stoked, noting that all calories were not created equal, which we have probably known all along on a logical level. The only thing constant is change and the "experts" advice will change as each diet craze runs its course. It is a multibillion dollar industry and always looking for something new and marketable even if it is an old idea in new packaging. This is why we must educate ourselves and we can do that through aligning our eating habits with our functioning.

The Purpose of Food

Let's refocus on the purpose of food. The role of food is not necessarily to taste good, but as you follow these principles you will find that your taste buds evolve, adapt and change to enjoy the food you are feeding it. The job of food is to provide fuel and building blocks to your body. Take your list of food you have eaten over the past few days and organize it into a scale. This is not about the micro or macro nutrient level, but based solely on how you felt shortly after consuming it. Start with the food that increases your energy level at the bottom, above it put any food that doesn't appear to have any effect on your state, and on top of that write down the food that takes your energy away. You will not have to run around writing everything you eat down for the rest of your life as some clear patterns will emerge. Hopefully through this you will begin to eat what energizes you more than what you are craving in the moment or desire emotionally. When you eat a meal that enhances your life you will start to function at a higher level. You will experience increased energy, mental acuity, and feel energized, happier and healthier. When you eat a meal that takes more energy to process than it provides you with, you will feel tired, your thought speed will slow and you will feel like some life has been taken from you. This is not the purpose of food.

Below is a food scale that energizes me and adds vitality to my life as an example for you to use while constructing your own scale. This will hopefully evolve into something you will use and add to your life to give more energy to your day.

Patterns will emerge. This is not rocket science and you probably already know what foods energize you and what takes away from you. If it comes through a drive thru chances are it is not going to energize you. If it is fresh, organic, local and alive most likely it will add more energy to your day. This is about what works for your life. Create that recipe to be in the state you want. Another way to note what the food will do is based on the nutrients it gives you versus the amount of energy it takes for your body to process it. Up to 70% of our bodies stress can come from our food. We can limit this stress by eating food that has high nutritional yield with low processing stress on our body. The more your body has to work to process the food the more nutrients you will need to gain from the food to make it worth while. Otherwise you are spending more energy on digestion than what the food gives you and therefore it is taking more life from you, than adding to you. Eating food that is local, natural, and organic often gives much more nutrients than it takes from you. The more processing of the food before it reaches your mouth, the more your body will need to process it for proper digestion and the more energy it takes from you versus supplying you with.

In this example food list, the food that takes energy from me is at the top, minimal impact food in the middle and the food that increases my energy level on the bottom.

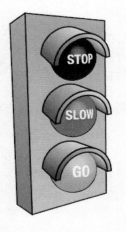

French fries

Potato Chips

Ice Cream

Coffee

Turkey Sandwich

Chicken

Almonds

Water

Apples

Peppers

Number them from 1 to 10.

1. French fries
2. Potato Chips
3. Ice Cream
4. Coffee
5. Turkey Sandwich
6. Chicken
7. Almonds
8. Water
9. Apples
10. Peppers

From 7 to 10, these are the green lists. Take the picture of a stop light, what drives you, what gets you going and gives life and vitality to your day? These are the green foods.

4 to 6 are the yellow foods. These are neutral, they neither take energy away nor add to it. These are the foods that have minimal impact on your state and you don't want to over do them, but don't need to be overly concerned about them. Some of these foods you may not feel any reaction to at this time, but might in the future depending on what activity you are doing at the time.

1 to 3 are the red foods, these are the energy drains. This is the red zone of your stoplight. These foods take energy from you and rob you of your vitality. This is the food that takes more energy to process than it gives you. These are the foods we often crave. They will fill our belly, but not help reach peak performance. These foods communicate lethargy and hibernation.

As you become your own expert you will start to eat according to how your body feels after the meal rather then how it feels in the moment in your mouth. Your tastes will adapt as change is the only constant. If you are used to eating fast foods, your body will crave those. If you are used to giving your body fresh fruits and vegetables, then your body will want more of that. Experiment with yourself and have fun. If you know what you should be eating, but are stuck eating through habits or from emotional reactions try not to focus on what you are not eating or taking out of your life. If you focus on limiting the red foods then you will only desire them more. Start by adding some green foods to your diet. If you eat a red food, pair it with a green and get used to adding green into your life. If you are going to eat some chocolate, have a strawberry with it. These small changes will add up over time. Take charge of what message you communicate to your body through your eating habits.

Sugar and Fat Cravings

A quick note on why your body craves sugar and fat. Early man foraging for food in the wild knew a berry was safe to eat by tasting it. They knew that if a food was sweet, it was good to eat, but if it was bitter it would make them sick. As for the cravings for sugar and fat this happens because they contain the highest density of calories out of any food source. It only takes a small amount of fat to give you the calories you need to keep from starving, whereas with protein and other carbohydrates you have to consume a much larger amount.

Movement and Energy

The second mode of communication with your body is through movement. This doesn't have to be about specific hours, minutes or type of exercise each day, this is about the overall message you are sending. This is about the lifestyle communication. What is the overall lifestyle message that you are telling your body to be prepared for? Is going to the gym for an hour then spending the rest of the day in bed as helpful as being active throughout the day walking, playing a sport or going for a swim? I'm not sure, only you can be the judge for yourself. I'm sure people on either side will argue for one or the other, or both. I know for me that the second choice is more sustainable, enjoyable and appears like a better, healthier life. It may not be that way for someone else, but I enjoy having an active day.

The next exercise is to create an energy scale based on what actions give and take energy from you. This is not related to emotions, we will cover that later on. Brainstorm some typical activities you do throughout the day. For example:

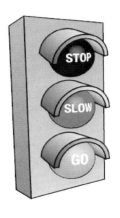

Activity Scale

1. Work drama
2. Argue with co-workers
3. Watch TV
4. Office gossip
5. Computer Work
6. Write
7. Walk
8. Hike
9. Jog
10. Play Hockey

Now take some time to organize some of your activities according to the red, yellow or green zones.

Your Personal Activity Scale

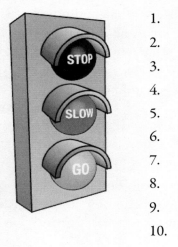

1.
2.
3.
4.
5.
6.
7.
8.
9.
10.

Consciously Communicate to Our Body

It is up to us individually to consciously communicate our needs to our body and take control of how we are operating ourselves. We need to increase our awareness of this message and how our fuel relates to our energy level and activity needs. We must tune into our fuel and energy systems.

Our physique is a reflection of how we communicate with the human reptile. At this level there is no thought, only instinct.

Therefore we have to send our body this communication through an instinctual means. This is by how we move, and the primary food we supply it with. This message is what is reflected through our lifestyle and our form we see in the mirror. It is up to us to take control with our higher brain functioning and operate this communication pathway to achieve maximum physical performance, rather than letting our genetics, or the environment control our functioning.

- How do you feel after you eat?

- What foods drain your energy? Energize you?

- Do you consciously link what you eat to what energy level you need to be at?

- What happens if you fuel yourself in a red zone, but need to have green energy?

- What activities move you into green? Yellow? Red?

- What energy level do you want to spend most of your day at?

- What do you need to do to be in the green zone?

- What is the relationship between food and how you are feeling?

- What message do you want to communicate to your body?

Briefcase Tools for Operating the Human Reptile

- Deep Breathe to manage the activating survival response

- Manage your state through posture control

- Tune into your fuel and energy systems

- Be your own expert and examine the relationship between food and energy

- To change your physical health you must change your communication through sending a different message of your lifestyle through fuel and movement

- To enhance processing of food take ten deep breaths before you eat to put yourself in a relaxing state to optimize digestion

Chapter 4

The Mammalian Brain

"We're animals. We're born like every other mammal and
we live our whole lives around disguised animal thoughts."

Barbara Kingsolver

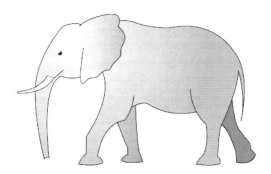

Emotional Overwhelm

Eight in the morning Cheryl greeted me at my office door with
tears streaming down her face. My lunch wasn't even unpacked yet
as her story came erupting out of her. She blurted out that she

couldn't take it anymore. He was late and she knew he was off cheating. Having only met her briefly once before, I was struggling to understand what she was talking about. I knew that when people are in emotional states they can get caught up in a cycle of emotional thinking where overwhelmed with emotions their stream of thoughts takes on a life of its own producing more emotional overwhelm. I could see that her thoughts and emotions were putting her into an extreme state activating her reptilian like survival mechanisms. Some of her symptoms were shallow breathing, increased heart rate, and her face looked flushed. I knew she had to take control of her inner reptile. I had to interrupt this cycle as she was spiralling out of control.

The easiest way to break patterned thinking is to bring someone into consciousness by doing something unexpected causing their brain to focus attention. So I smashed my coffee mug against the wall. I didn't really, but see how well it works! I bet I caught your attention. Anyways, I simply offered her my almond butter on Ezekiel bread sandwich from my unpacked lunch. In the moment she paused to process what I said before stating "no thank-you" and I quickly asked her to breathe with me. Knowing that in 5 to 10 deep breathes the reptilian's activating system is shut off putting her into the calming system. Here the reptiles focus is no longer getting blood and oxygen to the muscles, allowing increased blood flow to the top part of the brain re-engaging her abilities to think and problem solve. This allowed her the opportunity to take control of her basic emotions. In this state she could share her story in a way I could understand it. She was a 43 year old female struggling with a history of broken and unstable relationships. It is possible that she fits the diagnostic criteria of borderline personality disorder, but it was a little premature to treat for that, however I would keep that suspicion in the back of my mind for now. Either way I knew she would benefit from an understanding of how her mammalian brain works.

Mammalian Brain

The mammalian brain is also known as the limbic system. Its important functions are basic emotions, motivation, learning and memory. The mammalian brain is fully developed at around age 2 and is incapable of logical thought. For our purposes here I include the visceral system in the body as the second level of functioning, building from the most basic level directed by the reptilian brain. The purpose of the visceral system is to protect us from internal threats such as viruses. This system includes the immune response, and metabolism. It includes the heart, lungs, liver, stomach- basically your guts. This is where our need for connection to the environment is as we are influenced by light, nature, and interactions with each other.

A few years ago there was a study published in the journal Neuroscience indicating that a team of researchers discovered a bacteria found in soil called mycobacterium vaccae. This bacterium increases serotonin production in the part of the brain that regulates mood. Serotonin is the neurotransmitter (brain chemical) that most anti-depressants work on and is also known to enhance immune function. Lack of exposure to this bacterium has been linked to an increased vulnerability to asthma and allergy. We expose ourselves to these bacteria by ingesting or inhaling them by gardening, eating root vegetables, and hiking in the woods. It is ironic that some have allergies to the very thing that provides a buffer to getting allergies.

The mammalian brain is composed of the nervous system, reward, and fear system. Housed in the mammalian brain are the hippocampus which is involved in learning and memory, the amygdala which is also known as the fear warehouse, and the nucleus accumbens which is important in reward and motivation. The nucleus accumbens is where the dopamine reward passageway is, and is important in addiction as this is where the pleasure originates.

When we are in emotional states like Cheryl we often make decisions from the mammalian brain. The problem with this is that there is no deeper processing or analysis of these decisions because our higher brain functions that make us human are at the neocortex. Again, the mammalian brain only develops to age two and does not have the capacity for logic. So when we make decisions they are coming from either pain, pleasure, or based on what we did in similar circumstances in the past that aided our survival. This may let us survive, but we will never thrive by making decisions at this level. If we are operating ourselves solely from this level we are capable of learning from past experience, can feel fear, pain, and want to gain pleasure, however, we have no capacity for logic. This lines us up for poor choices that ultimately lead to more emotional discomfort and move us further away from having the great life we all deserve. Let's take a deeper look at our motivation system.

The Pain and Pleasure Principle of Motivation

Motivation in the mammalian brain works on a pain and pleasure principle. We seek to avoid pain and gain pleasure. Our drive to avoid pain is stronger than our drive to seek pleasure. Used together this comprises our motivational system. The pull for so many towards drugs and alcohol is strong as drugs give us immediate pain relief while producing pleasure. Drug and alcohol counselors are taught to use a strategy called motivation interviewing to help their clients address their substance use difficulties. Motivational strategies are applied to the client to basically, increase pain and reduce the pleasure associated with using drugs and alcohol. This is somewhat limiting as these strategies are applied to increase client motivation, but they do not go far enough in actually teaching a person how to operate their motivational system. What happens when a person is in need of motivational assistance outside of office hours? Hopefully, they have been taught to take control and operate their motivation system by learning how to use the pain and pleasure principle.

The cornerstone technique of motivational interviewing is a strategy called the decisional balance. This is basically a pro and con list that changes the short term associations of drug and alcohol use to a longer term, bigger picture outlook that essentially drums up the pain associated with substance use and decreases the experience of pleasure from the substance.

People involved in AA (alcoholics anonymous) and NA (narcotic anonymous) often talk about change happening as a result of experiencing the state of "rock bottom." This is thought of as the pinnacle moment of change, when things cannot get any worse and anything other than change is not a possibility. Essentially, the immediate short term gain of using, in that it takes away the pain and gives us pleasure, switches place with the longer term picture, where the drug or alcohol becomes more painful and less pleasurable than life without it. In a nutshell, the balance is shifted.

The long term picture is more real in the moment than the short term satisfaction of use. This is a long term view as the pain of using finally outweighs the pain that is taken away from use. The balance is shifted and the association of use is to the pain rather than the reward.

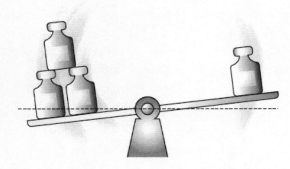

	Pain	Pleasure
Drug & alcohol use (short term)	Decreases	Increases
Hits rock bottom		
Long term view of use	Increases	Decreases

Most drug and alcohol dependent people never plan on moving all their possession into shopping carts this happens through the habituation process while operating from the mammalian brain. The pain and pleasure principle is applicable to all human behaviors. An example of this is with procrastinators.

Procrastination

When we procrastinate, the pain associated with doing the activity combined with the pleasure of not doing the activity, is more real and powerful, than the pleasure of accomplishing the activity combined with the pain of not having it done.

Procrastinator	Pain	Pleasure
Doing the activity (short term)	Increased	Decreased
Stopping procrastination means focus of having the activity done (long term)	Decreased	Increased

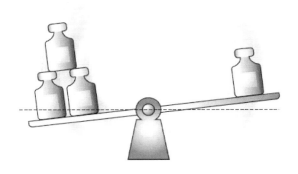

It is your choice how you operate your motivation system. In university, for tests and term papers I waited until the last possible moment before completing the paper or studying for exams. I was often writing or studying under the feeling of extreme pressure and up very late at night. I waited until the pain was so intense that not doing the paper meant the ultimate pain, failure. At this point, I could do nothing else but get the paper done. My friend Lindsay was the opposite. First week of school she would start her research and a month into the semester she would have her term paper done. Over the next three months she was stress free and would revise her work as she pleased. Needless to say she always got better grades. What was real for her was that the pain of putting the work into it immediately paid off in the pleasure of being done and not having to worry about it for the next three months.

The Key to Our Motivational System

We can control our motivational system by using this strategy. The key is to drum up the pain and pleasure on an emotional level. Knowing that it is the middle part of our brain with our basic emotions that we use if we want to stop procrastinating, and I assume that you want to stop procrastinating, requires a shift in the balance between your current behavior and what you want to stop procrastinating about. For example, if I was to operate myself differently at university I would first need a time machine and second I would need to ask myself some different questions. Instead of focusing on everything else that I could do in the moment, I could focus on how good I will feel when I have my term paper done, and how painful it would be to spend the rest of the semester knowing I had this term paper to do in the back of my mind. The important piece is to operate your self on an emotional level, the more intense the better.

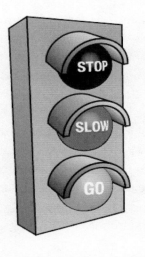

Emotions Scale

Now let's look at an emotions scale:

1. Shame
2. Guilt
3. Apathy
4. Grief
5. Anger
6. Optimism
7. Acceptance
8. Peace
9. Love
10. Joy

Picture a corresponding traffic control light with the top being the red emotions or your painful moving away emotions, while your green is moving towards or pleasure emotions, and the yellow is the in between emotions or neutral.

Now take a couple of minutes and construct your own scale.

Your Personal Emotions Scale

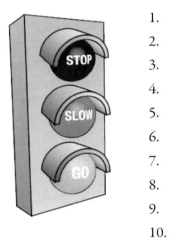

1.

2.

3.

4.

5.

6.

7.

8.

9.

10.

The green zone is moving towards emotions, these are also your pleasurable emotions. Red are the painful emotions and also your moving away from emotions. This emotion scale acts like a warning system. Emotions should not solely dictate your behavior. You are not operated by your emotions; you are in control of them. Through this scale you can control your motivation, memory, anxiety, etc.

Taking control of the mammalian brain goes further to ensure success than any other change you can make. This is where the negative voice that undermines you is located and is where fear begins. This is where the filter that can take docile information and turn it into a threat that you over react to. Or this is where you can choose not to react. To filter negative information out, tell yourself that you are safe and it's okay to take chances. What moves you into green, or red? Can you control the state you are in? How do you do this?

Basic Emotions are not higher brain functions, they are a reflex. These are emotions we experience before we get to think about the situation and process with the neocortex. In the mammalian brain, emotions work as a guidance system for us, they give us feedback. They let us know if we are safe, on track or off track, and allow us to move toward energy versus drain our energy. What happens when you are angry? This emotion system can work as a warning system if we pay attention to the message we are feeling. Are the majority of your emotions moving towards (green), or moving away emotions (red)? What color are you in right now?

Cheryl in the Red Zone

In Cheryl's case she was living in the red zone. Her actions were designed to move her out of pain, but as she was not processing at a higher brain level she inevitably set herself up for more pain. Cheryl lived in such a strong survival state that the mere thought of moving towards a pleasurable life was so foreign to her, that when I brought it up she recoiled in fear. I had planted a seed though, and for now that was enough. She was living based on her reflex emotions, in a state of fear. In time she would start to monitor what color she was in. Using emotions as a monitoring system she began to take control and if she started to be in red, she would deep breathe and take time to think things through instead of reacting. If she was in green, she learned that she was on track and would do more of what was working. This small step began to pay massive dividends in her life. Instead of jumping to the conclusion that if he was late, he was cheating on her, she learned to deep breathe and calm her inner reptile and the associated survival mechanisms, allowing her to think from a higher level. She learned to recognize when thoughts were streaming from the fear warehouse in the mammalian brain and knew its function was to keep her safe, but it would never let her take the risk of having a healthy relationship where she was vulnerable and trusting. Cheryl would step back, breathe and consider other alternatives as to why he may be late. This set the stage to reduce some of the conflict that would inevitably drive her partners out of her life. The emotional reflex is initially processed by what information is drawn in through our senses, but first it has to pass through our filter.

Filter

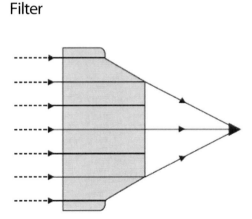

The Fear Warehouse

The filter is in the mammalian brain where it communicates directly with the amygdala, which is known as the fear warehouse. Our filter strains the information collected from the environment by our senses to identify what is relevant to us. Survival is given priority over all else. The actual part of the brain that is mainly responsible for this filtering process is called the Reticular Activating System or RAS. The RAS is the center where the information from the external world collected by the senses meets the information from the internal world, mostly from the neocortex. This is the point where the external and internal world converges. Here information is passed along to the amygdala and from the amygdala to the rest of the brain, either up to the neocortex for complex processing or down to the motor cortex of the reptilian brain to move and take action. The RAS has no intelligence and cannot differentiate between thought and reality. When information is passed along to the amygdala, which determines based on past information whether we are safe or not, the amygdala does not know if the tiger it is reacting to is a thought, or reality. This is how our thoughts can trigger panic attacks, or a feeling of safety in an unsafe environment. The RAS will scan for information that corresponds to the thoughts we are thinking. The RAS is essential to learning, motivation, attention, and self-control.

Information is collected by our senses filtered through the RAS and processed by the amygdala to determine if we are safe or not. This determination is made based on past experience of what has happened in similar circumstances. If we are safe the sensory information is passed along to the neocortex for more complex processing. If the amygdala determines we are not safe then it tells the body to mobilize, turning on our protection system. This is why you can never completely let go of the past as it serves a survival function. If you get mugged while walking through a dark alley at night you will never completely let go of the memory associated with that event. Nor should you as the fear is there to keep you safe. Some remain in the fear state too long and their amygdala becomes hot-wired for fear. This over activity of the amygdala is also known as a "hot-amygdala" and is associated with anxiety, depression, post traumatic stress disorder and other maladies. This can be decreased by maintaining a low level of arousal while having experiences that contradict the fear message.

In times of great stress, anxiety, depression, or extreme emotional states our filter can become overloaded by sensorial stimuli. The volume of stimulus becomes so great that information normally filtered out seeps through causing overwhelm or an overloaded feeling. In these times you can reset the filter by moving to environments where there is less stimulation, such as lying in bed or going to a quiet dark place, or by sleeping. A colleague of mine works on a specialized adolescent psychiatric unit and has observed this phenomenon in children who are experiencing psychosis. She asserts that when these kids are in a psychotic state they need to reset themselves which is done by a standard method of treatment of sleep and de-stimulation.

This is a common experience for people where the need to reset the filter may present itself as anxiety, depression, or even migraine headaches. Most people with migraines become hyper sensitive to light, noise and movement and need to lie down in a dark bedroom until the pain passes. I had a psychology professor in university tell us a story of his physician giving him some strong medication for his migraines. He started to track when he gets the pain and noticed that it was around times of high stress, or when he was neglecting to take proper care of himself. He also recognized that every time his spouse's parents were visiting them with their small pack of poodles and endless noise, a migraine was triggered. He would take some pain killers, lie down in his quiet bedroom and fall asleep, waking up to an empty low stimulation house and he would feel better.

Another common way to deal with an over flowing filter is to drink alcohol or use drugs. A lot of people with anxiety disorders use this strategy. Obviously, it does not allow them to learn to deal with their anxiety or control it in a healthy manner as the alcohol or drugs provide a numbing effect to the filter. It does not fix the problem, but decreases the activity of the neocortex, lowers brain function and reduces the amount of stimulus that the brain is able to sense, filter and process. When we spend a lot of time in an activating state it is necessary to consciously give yourself a break and allow the filter to reset itself before you return to activation mode. To do this you need to calm the reptile by deep breathing, putting yourself in a growth state and finding a safe place with a low level of distraction and noise to take a break. Life is not an endurance sport; it is a series of sprints and recovery zones. When we are in high stress and activated for a long time, we must balance playing hard with resting hard.

Unloading an Overloaded Filter

Counseling can be effective to get you into a calming state, help you process information, and file it away in order to help reset your filter. When a filter becomes over stimulated by trauma, abuse, or emotional over-load, sitting down and processing the information to reduce your sensitivity to it can be very helpful. As long as you are not increasing the reaction by endlessly reliving the event, as this is not beneficial and sets people up to remain in a fear state.

You can implant messages into your filter through the RAS.

This is also a part of the reframing process of counseling. When something happens in our environment we react to it based on our previous experience. However we can change the meaning of an event by reframing, or changing the tint of our filter. A client I had complained of reacting every time her husband slammed the kitchen cupboards shut. To her this represented anger and was an avenue to passive-aggressively push her buttons. When she sat back and processed where this was coming from she realized that she was reacting the way her mother did to her father. She also identified that she didn't have the type of relationship with her husband that her parents had. At home, she asked her husband why he slammed the cupboards, something that he did not even know he was doing. From then on he agreed to be more mindful of the force he uses to close the cupboards. We can affect the tint of our filter through the messages we give ourselves about what something represents, or what we are expecting to happen. This is why positive affirmations work.

Why Affirmations Work

Positive affirmations work because the RAS can not differentiate synthetic reality from reality perceived through your senses. If you see a tiger coming at you, your fear reaction activates putting you into fight, flight or freeze mode. Your RAS filters out all information except for the tiger and sends it to the amygdala which signals the survival mechanisms to respond. As the RAS cannot differentiate between a real threat of a tiger from negative self-talk, the fear system activates in both circumstances. A tiger will draw a more immediate and serious response as the threat is much greater. If you worked hard you could work yourself into the same reaction with your thoughts, but it may take a little longer than if you fell into a tiger cage.

If you are approaching a group of people and your fear response is activated as you are expecting a negative reaction, you are more likely to have a bad experience as your RAS sensitizes towards information to follow its expectation. This is why we have self fulfilling prophecies as we become sensitive to certain stimuli and in this case it is looking for information to back up the state of fear. You walk up to the group bracing your self with your expectation for criticism, filled with fear and physically bent over appearing in a non-responsive state. Even neutral stimuli will be perceived as threatening as the filter is tinted with fear. Conversely just the opposite is true, if you are expecting that people will like you or are thinking that you have a great story to tell the group then you will physically appear positive and your RAS will be filtering for information that backs up this different mind set. A person making eye contact will be seen as interest rather than as a threat or attempt to intimidate. It is a whole different reality.

Your filter looks for the information to back up its expectation and triggers the physiological response just as it would with stimulus external to you. Instead of seeing the tiger outside and triggering the fear response, you trigger it internally with your thoughts. Because the mammalian brain developed before the neocortex it is not conscious of the existence of it. The mammalian brain works without logic and feeds it information it does not have the ability of the neocortex to analyze, think critically and question. Instead it reacts and can contribute to you living in an emotionally over reactive state. Affirmations work as you are feeding that part of your brain that does not question or think with logic, information that sends a different message.

You are using the neocortex to send a message through the RAS that you are safe, brilliant and competent. This message is passed along which calms the amygdala and out to the rest of the mammalian and reptilian brain causing a physiological response that puts you in a positive state and begins a chain reaction that works for you, instead of undermining you. All this can be summed up with the statement that our body reacts the same way from thoughts about stress as it does to real stress. The same is true for encouraging thoughts, and fearful ones.

Fear System

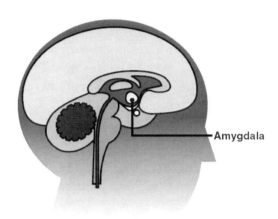

Amygdala

Fear and Our Physiological Survival Mechanisms

The fear system is what has helped us survive for thousands of years and is one of the most basic and universal of all human traits. The problem is that our society has changed so much in the last hundred years that we no longer need to be concerned with day to day survival, yet we have this hard wired fear system. This fear system developed to react to external, concrete threats such as a tiger chasing us, but is also activated by abstract stimulus such as excessive emails, bills, and financial problems. With either the concrete or abstract stimulus the same physiological survival mechanisms react. Stress hormones are released into the blood stream and our chemical composition is altered. This happens whether the stress is a thought or real in our environment.

The amygdala is where these internal fear messages originate from that undermine our sense of confidence and ability to take risks. It is that little voice in your head that tells you not to take risks like public speaking, or answering a question in school despite knowing the correct response. It does this for a reason and that is to achieve safety. If you don't take any risks you will not look foolish, or feel embarrassed. At this level it is all about safety. The amygdala gives us those messages that the world is a big dark scary place and we would be better off lying in bed. The same chemical release and physical reaction happens when you are afraid of getting embarrassed or risking the chance of injury. However you cannot live a fulfilling life while lying in bed with the covers pulled over your head.

We are able to shut down the fear response of the amygdala by first shutting down the inner reptile which we do by deep breathing. Second, research has shown that by putting yourself in a state of gratitude, appreciation, or love results in decreased blood flow to the amygdala or fear warehouse. Decreased blood flow, means decreased oxygen, which results in less fuel to the fear warehouse. By putting yourself in a state of appreciation, love or gratitude you essentially decrease the fear messages that emanate from your mammalian brain. Take this scenario as an example.

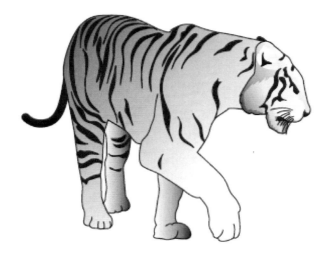

You walk down the street, the bushes rustle and a tiger jumps out. Depending on its trajectory, distance from you and general attitude you are either going to fight, flight or freeze. When the danger passes and the tiger is no where around you, your heart rate lowers, your amygdala determines you are safe and you can continue on your day. The next day you are in the same place and your amygdala is on high alert, the normal scanning of the environment that you do will be heightened and brought into conscious awareness. If the bushes rustle your survival mechanisms will kick in and you will run away without even seeing a tiger jump out. Three days before, you may not have even reacted to the bushes rustling, most likely passing it off as the wind. This is the survival mechanisms that developed to keep early man safe and is still with us today, despite our society being safe, no matter what picture the news may paint for us. We do not have to concern ourselves with dinosaur attacks when we are at the local grocery store.

Nervous System

We work from one of two nervous systems. The first is the parasympathetic nervous system or calming system, the second is the sympathetic nervous system or activating system. The calming system is a growth system, while the activating system is built for protection. In growth, blood flows to the top part of our brain or neocortex. Our body uses fat as the primary fuel source and the body develops and repairs itself. Digestion is maximized as the body's relaxation response is activated. The body has full metabolic force and produces energy. The hypothalamus pituitary adrenal axis (HPA) is inactive which I will discuss later on. Finally, there is increased blood to the visceral system and neocortex which enhances digestion and intelligence.

The protection system is operated from the mammalian and reptilian brain. The mammalian brain tells the reptilian brain when to jump into protection mode. In protection, carbohydrates are the primary fuel source resulting in carbohydrate cravings as the body wants quick fuel to use in activation. The body desires quick energy to maintain safety through short bursts of activity such as sprinting to safety. Growth is suppressed and digestion is turned off. Blood flows to the musco-skeletal system for protection. Alertness is increased as well as strength. Information is processed at a faster rate and the fight, flight, or freeze reflex is engaged. There is decreased blood flow to the neocortex as a result higher brain functions are reduced as they are not essential for survival. The body's energy reserves are depleted as resources are drained to survive. We actually lose intelligence in this state and this is often the reason why people do out of character things while angry, such as assaulting someone. The stress hormones adrenaline and cortisol are released. These increase strength and speed, but cause fat to be stored and prevent muscle growth while in this state. Blood flow to the skeletal muscles and lungs is enhanced by up to 1200%. Oxygen exchange and transport is enhanced as well as heart rate. Pupils dilate as senses become more acute.

This is how Cheryl presented in my office that day and it soon became clear that she was living in this state most of the time. As she began to understand her difficulties this set the stage for her to learn to take better control of how she was operating herself. She argued that she was not in control of her functioning and her strong feelings of being out of control convinced her of this. I knew that if she could start to accept that she was in control of these biological functions then she would began to consciously take some of that control back.

If we continue in a prolonged protection state for too long our body becomes malnourished as nutrients are not evenly distributed, we have hormonal imbalances, anxiety, sleep disturbances and depression. This is due to a shrinking hippocampus and prefrontal cortex as the body is over stressed.

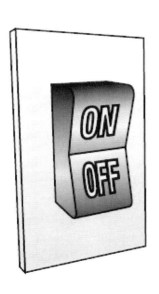

Which system do you work from most of the time? In growth or protection? What does that do to your body? How does this effect performance? Our goal should be to consciously spend more time in growth than protection. How do you drive home from work, in growth or protection? When people eat food on the run their body is in protection mode. This doesn't allow all the nutrients to get properly processed as the digestive system is shut down and cortisol signals the body to store fat.

Switching from Protection to Growth

As mentioned in the last chapter you can switch from protection mode to growth by taking five to ten deep diaphragmatic breathes. Deep breathing calms the reptile and allows you to move back into the calming system. Taking ten deep breaths before you eat switches your body into the state of growth, activating your full metabolic and digestive force. This enables you to fully process the food and extract the maximum amount of nutrients available and evenly distribute them to your body. In this state your body maintains and repairs itself increasing your health rather than depleting its resources for safety. Aside from eating, calming your reptile through deep breathing also decreases anxiety and symptoms of stress. Deep breathing can be used anywhere without people knowing. You can use it before writing a test, in the line at the bank, or before a meal with complete confidentiality. Traditional European ways of eating naturally incorporate this into their culture around meals. This is evidenced by the French paradox.

The French paradox comes from the observation that the French suffer a relatively low incidence of coronary heart disease, despite having a diet that is high in saturated fats. In 1991 it was suggested that this was due to the large amount of red wine that they consume, arguing that red wine decreases the incidence of cardiac diseases. The consumption of red wine in North America increased 44%. Further studies indicated that it was more due to the relationship the French have with food and how they use it in their culture. Their process of eating often lasts an hour or more as they socialize, savor their food and unwittingly deep breathe. What is your relationship with food? Do you often eat on the run?

HPA Axis

There is a second protection switch called the HPA axis. This switches us from our internal mammalian immune system response that fights infection, to our reptilian external fight/flight or freeze mechanism. Transplant doctors prescribe stress hormones for surgery to activate the body's fight, flight and freeze response as it turns off immune function so foreign tissue is not rejected during surgery. This works the way it does to enhance survival. For example, your body is fighting an infection and you are lying in bed with a fever, suddenly that tiger from the bushes, leaps through your window and onto your bed. In an instant your mammalian response is shut off and your reptilian survival mechanism is turned on. You either run to safety or fight it off until it jumps back through the window. When your mammalian brain determines that you are safe again, your immune response will return and your body will heat up to fight the infection.

The mammalian brain is more advanced than the reptilian but we still need to take control of how we operate it. When we are in an emotional state we can take ten deep breathes to calm the reptile and remove our self from the protection state. Food that has been eaten in a fear state gets processed differently than food eaten in a pleasure state. Eating on the go simulates the fear state and therefore the food that we consume does not get processed properly. You need to consciously use the pain/pleasure principle to operate your motivation system, and use your emotions as your guidance system to let you know if you are on track of not. Finally put your self in a state of gratitude, appreciation, or love to quiet the fear based voice of the amygdala, and allow your higher brain functions to activate.

Briefcase Tools for Operating your Inner Mammal

- Deep breathe to calm the reptile

- Put yourself in a state of gratitude, appreciation, or love

- Give yourself breaks to reset the filter

- Spend more time in the calming growth system than in protection

- Eat in a growth state

- Send positive thoughts to your filter to perceive the world in a positive light

- Motivate yourself with the pain and pleasure principle

- Use your emotional guidance system to know if you are on track

Chapter 5

The Neocortex

"It stands to the everlasting credit of science that by acting on the human mind it has overcome man's insecurity before himself and before nature."

Albert Einstein

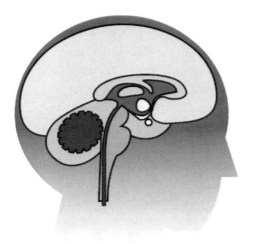

Jack's Pain

Jack was struggling with anxiety, depression and a crack cocaine addiction. He entered my office ready to give up and stated that he has been trying to quit using for over ten years, with no success. In that time, the longest he was able to stay away from using was at most a couple of weeks. His wife left him, his kids wouldn't speak to him, he had lost his job, his housing, everything he ever cared about, but still he could not quit. He said he hit rock bottom countless times and every time he thought he had nothing left to lose, somehow he would find a way to drive something else out of his life. He was desperate to change, but still his use persisted.

Jack was speaking to me on a logical level, I could see that his talk had become clichéd and meaningless. This often happens to people who attend countless meetings and learn the talk and belief system of some self help groups. After a certain amount of time hearing the same stories and the same rules to being an addict, the meaning dissolves leaving behind a defeatist psychology that at best is meaningless and at worst sets someone up for a lot more failure. This was the case with Jack and as he had so much counseling over the years that perpetuated his cycle of struggle, it was time to hit him from a different angle. A lot of counselors get into the field to help people. They are uncomfortable with another's suffering and want to help take their pain away. This may be coming from a caring place, but sets people up for failure because what they need at the motivational level is more suffering. Family systems often fall peril to this as they try to shield their drug or alcohol dependent family member from the pain of their consequences and essentially help them maintain their problem.

I once worked with a young man who every time he ran up a big tab with his drug dealer, his mother, again from a place of caring, would run down and pay off the dealer so he wouldn't hurt her son. Her actions make sense on a caring, logical level, but in the bigger picture she was only improving her son's credit rating with his drug dealer. The dealer also knew that someone was there to rescue her son and cover the tab. If you pay off your credit card a few times, the banks raise your limit. Same holds true for drug dealers. Counselors do the same thing, in an effort to help and suppress pain, they often cause more, and this is especially true in the drug and alcohol field. What Jack needed was massive pain. Jack learned all the skills he needed to deal with triggers or cope with cravings, what he was missing was complete and utter misery. The pain was already in his life, but he dealt with it by pushing it away or running out to smoke crack. He needed to hold off his negative coping strategies that seek to suppress pain, and feel the misery on the mammalian level. This would increase his motivation and make anything less than change, simply not enough. The difficult part is keeping him from running out to use as you start to amplify his pain. Also, it becomes counterproductive if he does not attend next session, or switches counselor. To enhance a person's pain you need to first have some rapport with them, and then you can help them face what everyone wants to avoid the most, suffering. I had him tell me how great his life would be if he did take a break from substance use. I always try to steer clear of having people say they will never use again as the rest of their life is too much to take on in the moment, when they are trying to go just one day without use. This often sets them up for failure before they even begin. When people commit to taking a break, set a short term goal and accomplish it, they discover that their life is so much better that they want to build on their success and they continue their break from use.

I'm not a masochist, but I do understand how the brain is structured and what is needed at each level. For Jack, he was functioning from a place that required massive pain and as I convinced him to allow himself to put down his guards and truly feel the pain, his motivation to make changes increased. This was the starting place he needed, but he had a long road before him. Now that he had some motivation, I had to teach him to change his beliefs that were so tightly ingrained in him, to break habits, and completely change how he was operating himself. He had to learn to take himself off automatic pilot and take conscious control of himself, despite having a theory that he had a disease that he would have for the rest of his life that is incurable.

Three Qualities of Psychologically Healthy People

Daniel Goleman who is famous for writing the emotional intelligence series of books wrote an article describing three essential qualities of psychologically healthy people. These people had hope, optimism, and a perception of control. Unfortunately, the addiction industry teaches people that they have a disease that they will have for the rest of their life, and that the only way to cope with this disease is to forego their power to something outside of themselves. This can be very counterproductive to helping people quit substance abuse. With an absence of hope no wonder people with substance use show such high rates of depression and failed attempts at quitting. Jack needed the opposite, he needed to understand how he functions, and that he could take control of this functioning and change how he operates himself. As the process of feeling the pain was increasing his motivation to change, the next step for him was a new education.

Successful Treatment is in the Neocortex

Despite addiction and many other disorders being based in the mammalian brain, the route to successful treatment is in the neocortex. The neocortex is the control panel of human operations. It is the conscious decision maker, the master of your functioning. The neocortex is the control panel that presents the opportunity to take us out of drug and alcohol dependency, anxiety, depression and personality disorders among others. It is the center that houses the "human spirit" and is essentially what makes us human. Humans have the largest neocortex of any other creature.

The neocortex is where we have our executive functions, language and creativity. Important in this is the brains ability to change, reorganize and rewire itself. Previously, scientists believed that the brain didn't change after a specific age but now they know that the brain is able to change. It is malleable or plastic. That is why we use the word neuroplasticity to describe the brain's ability to change. In the plasticity of the brain is where we develop habits and neuromaps.

A neuromap is basically a cluster of connections, organized around certain events, behaviors, thoughts, or feelings. Its purpose is to increase efficiency and decrease energy output when doing repetitive things. This is the basis of habit formation and why we have that feeling of automatic pilot after doing something we have done 791 times before. This is great news for people who are trying to break a habit or create a new life. You can change the way your brain wires information together.

Key Features of the Neocortex or Human Mind

Executive Functions

planning   flexibility   inhibition   anticipation

critical evaluation   working memory   abstract thinking

divided attention   decision making   goalsetting

foresight   cost/benefit analysis   language   creativity

Neuroplasticity

Jack's drug use had created neuroplastic changes in his brain that if left alone would continue to be reinforced and made bigger by continued substance abuse. To help him create some significant changes he needed to understand the concept of neuroplasticity and that it is possible to rewire his brain and change his drug dependency.

Neuroplasticity is the new frontier of science. It is the brain's ability to reorganize itself by forming new neuronal connections. A neuron is a cell that is specific to brain functioning. When we learn something new or install a habit, we form new connections between cells in the brain. Historically, scientists believed that our brains were fixed at around age 18 and developed very little if at all after that. This belief persisted and until as little as 15 to 20 years ago. Then a breakthrough discovery occurred that showed not only is the brain not fixed, but it changes throughout the lifespan creating a need for a radical shift in how we teach our clients.

Take for example piano players. The brain is divided down the middle and separated into a right and a left hemisphere which communicate with one another through a network of fibers known as the corpus callosum. Research into piano players, indicates that they have increased communication between the two hemispheres, most likely as a result of their ability to play the piano. Playing the piano requires playing separate notes by each hand at the same time in coordination with the other side of the brain. The left hemisphere controls the right side of the body while the right hemisphere controls the left side of the body. When we are playing the piano these two sides must be in harmony with the other. The not so simple act of learning to play the piano has the by-product of teaching the hemispheres of the brain to communicate more effectively with each other. This is important if you are planning on having some brain injury as it makes it easier for the brain to compensate between the hemispheres if one side is having a problem and needing the other to pick up the slack. By learning to play the piano, you have rewired and reorganized how your brain functions. Every time you master something new, whether it be the piano or learning what the word of the day is, a new connection is formed and you effectively have changed your brain. This can create problems with negative habits and behaviors such as with Jack; however this also allows us to make changes to how we are operating ourselves and rewire our brain in positive directions.

Dolphin Boy

There is no greater example of the potential of neuroplasticity than the life of Ben Underwood. Around age two, Ben lost his eyesight and with the love and support of his family he learned early on to not let his life be limited by his disability. Ben learned the skill of self-reliance as he felt his way around the world. His family helped him not by putting socks on his feet if they were cold, but by teaching him how to feel the seams to make sure the heal was on correctly, something I still struggle with! Ben began making clicking noises with his mouth and over time discovered how to tell where stationary objects were in his environment based on how the vibrations came back to him. Like a kind of human sonar much like dolphins use, he found his way around the world. He was completely blind, but he could bike, skate, climb trees, and even play video games. Ben passed away on January 19, 2009, seven days before his seventeenth birthday, but his life serves as a message to all of us about human adaptability and the amazing potential of humans.

Neuromaps and Habits

Ben made incredible neuroplastic changes reorganizing his brain's ability to process sight and enabled himself to push the limits of human capacity by developing the skill of echolocation. Jack was on the other side of the spectrum using his brain's capacity to wire in negative habits that set him up to struggle with life. When we make connections between behaviors over and over again they develop into a kind of file for the brain that pairs associated behaviors together. Over time this forms a type of neuromap.

Central to the brain's ability to process complex tasks simultaneously is the need for efficiency. It is through this need for efficiency that we create habits. When we do things repetitively we no longer need to focus as much energy on the task. Have you ever arrived at home from work and wondered how you got there? Unsure if you put yourself at risk or not because you feel like you had not paid any attention to your driving. This is because through repetitive experience the brain begins to create maps. These neuromaps are the basis of habits. Ivan Pavlov, a famous scientist, discovered that if he rang a bell when presenting a dog with food enough times causing the dog to salivate, then he could instigate further salivation by ringing the bell without the presentation of food. This is known as paired association. The dog's brain learned that bell ringing meant incoming food and became organized into a map in the dog's brain.

Neuromap in Action

When you drive to your new job on the first day you may need to read road signs, look for parking, and maybe feeling nervous about what's to come on your first day. You need a lot of conscious attention to make sure you get to the right place and be on time. When its day 792 at the same job and you know what to expect, you know how to get there and could park with your eyes closed, you do not need much conscious awareness to complete the task of getting to work on time. Your focus of attention is reduced as you do not need very much energy to complete the task. Your brain as an efficient machine cannot afford to waste energy doing something so mindless. So in the morning when you head to your car, the brain opens the "get to work" file. If during the trip a ball rolls out in front of you or something unexpected happens, you are instantaneously brought back to conscious awareness and can make the necessary adjustments. If you need to stop for milk, or change your routine in anyway, your brain will focus more attention on the task, or you will surely forget the milk.

I worked with a woman named Victoria who was trying to reduce her alcohol use. She had installed a habit of every time she went to the grocery store she would hit the liquor store next door. Outside of her trips for grocery's she was doing excellent, but every time she went for grocery's she came home with alcohol. She would report that she would either be in the store making the purchase, in her car, or sometimes even at home before she would realize what she was doing. I chuckled when she used the phrase "it's like I'm on automatic pilot." It's true, she was on automatic pilot. She was following a map that she had installed with little conscious attention. After discussing this with her she came up with a few different strategies to keep her attention when grocery shopping. On her next two sessions she reported that her strategies worked. She always parked on the same side of the lot in between the liquor and grocery store. Instead she parked on the opposite side. She shopped at a different grocery store a couple of times, and drove a different way to the original grocery store. These simple strategies required enough conscious attention that it kept her off automatic pilot and operating herself from the neocortex rather than the mammalian brain.

Love is a prime example of a complex neuromap that resembles an addiction map and the following story brings it to life.

Neuromap of Love

"Neurons that fire together wire together"

The human brain is constantly changing, developing and updating its systems and structure. As we experience life both internally and externally we engage in our own neurological evolution. The brain changes that occur through learning and living roughly follow this simplified pattern. Connections form between two relatively independent cells in the brain or neurons. As cells fire together and wire more complex connections form.

These more complex systems bind together to form a

neurological representational or neuromap. Neuromaps change and evolve as new connections form or old connections dissolve. This is a form of neuroplasticity. Maps or links need to be reinforced to be maintained or over time they will dissolve allowing the space to be used more efficiently. Much like if no one drives on a dirt road for a long time it becomes overgrown by the surrounding vegetation.

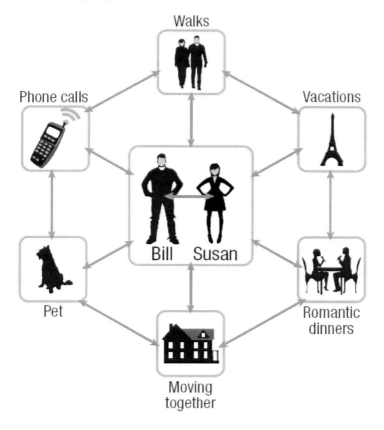

Bill and Susan meet. They fall in love as they spend excessive amounts of time together experiencing each other and the world.

Chris Douglas

They do all the things new lovers do. They spend time together, go to movies, talk on the phone, and can't keep their hands off each other. Every Saturday night they go to dinner, walk on the beach then go to a movie together thus creating a mini-representational subsystem within the larger map called "date night." They move in together, share toothpaste, find a new pasta sauce that they both can agree on and set up their friends David and Shelly who go on to create there own neuromap under the title of "relationship." Their lives and neuromaps become reinforced as they move in together, invest in a small apartment size animal, and purchase matching track suits that they may or may not wear to the mall together. Their living neuromap of their life together continues to grow and develop. There is routine, habit and a deep sense of connection.

One day Bill gets a new job as a traveling salesman. He is gone for long periods of time and they miss each other. It is all very sad, but very beautiful. Bill heads into the mountains and has no phone coverage limiting contact between the two. The withdrawal symptoms begin and their physical symptoms are similar to what drug and alcohol dependent people go through. They get butterflies in their stomach, can't eat, and are experiencing a rollercoaster of emotions from "I miss him/her so much," to "everything's going to be all right we'll be together soon." Then suddenly on the four hundred and twenty second attempt, Bill's phone gets through and they talk for hours. They're relieved and elated. Bill finishes his trip and they are re-united. Life is good. The neuromap is reinforced and they both feel better, they had their fix. As Bill's trips become a regular occurrence a new map may develop called "Bill away."

Bill being the shrewd salesman that he is, sold so much in the mountains that he is named salesman of the year and given a bonus cruise in the Caribbean sea. Unfortunately, Susan cannot attend, but given that she is a trusting, emotionally healthy woman, she

90

urges Bill to go without her. Bill pressured by the company executives and dire need for a sun tan, he reluctantly accepts. Hugs, kisses, Hawaiian shirts and a lengthy wave from Susan send Bill off on his cruise, to return in two weeks.

Tragedy strikes, the ship is lost in the Bermuda triangle and never heard from again. Bill is dead. Susan is distraught and goes through the stages of grief, which are denial, anger, bargaining, depression, and acceptance. Now, not everyone goes through these stages and not necessarily in order, but the most important one is the last. To risk being boring, and taking the romance out of the beautiful part of this story I will tell you what happens in the brain. What happens to the neuromap is that Susan now has this map that no longer fits her reality. Had Bill been a goldfish it is possible she could have just bought a new one and named it Bill 2.

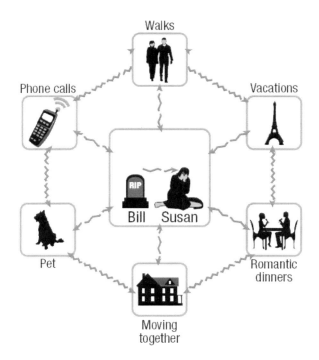

However, he is human and not easily replaced.

On to the stages of grief and first up is denial. "Bill is not dead, he can't be." Essentially she is saying "I have this neuromap of him that clearly shows him as part of my life and therefore he is alive, I have a neurological representational map of him.'

Next is anger. "Bill's not dead; I hate you for telling me that." This of course loosely translates into "how dare you say my neuromap no longer fits reality."

Third is bargaining. "If you bring Bill back I will never lie, cheat or eat chocolate ever again," which means "please, let my neuromap be real, I'll do anything, its too difficult letting it go."

On to depression, Susan lies in bed, she can't eat, doesn't go outside, she again is having those withdrawal symptoms we experience when we need to reorganize our brain and dissolve a neuromap that no longer fits our reality. Her self talk at this stage translates into "it's very sad to let a neuromap go, I don't want to live without it." She lies in bed clutching a picture of him tightly to her chest. Thus, firing her neuromap of life with Bill in an attempt to reinforce the map and keep it in the system. However the next stage follows close behind.

Finally acceptance hits, and in acceptance a neuromodulator is released as it is official, her map no longer fits the territory. Susan is now ready to move on. She puts away the pictures that were causing her grief to be prolonged, and takes over his side of the closet. He is finally dead to her. She reasons that he is gone, and she misses him, but they had a good run and with Bill being roughly the same size as her, she doubled her wardrobe.

Neuromodulators enhance or diminish synaptic connections. They wipe our learned behavior, and make room for new attachments. In this case Bill is removed from Susan's wiring. He stays as a memory of her life, but is no longer wired into the neuromap of daily life. Susan has broken the habit of Bill. She has gone through her withdrawal symptoms, stages of grief and neuromodulators are released dissolving the connections. These chemicals are powerful and with them come an endorphin like state and a feeling that "everything is going to be all right." This chemical produces the feeling of acceptance and boosts mood.

Days later, after that feeling of acceptance, Susan bumps her grocery cart into Johnny and their eyes lock. Its love at first sight and now that she has room in her brain to create a new neuromap the process starts all over again. Johnny and her go to the movies, talk on the phone, and walk the dog that recently dissolved his neuromap of life with Bill as well.

Neuromap of love

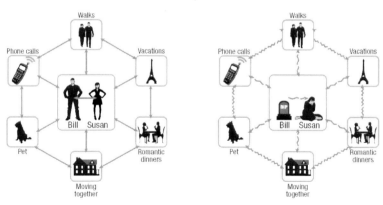

Erasing a Map

Installing a map takes time and this is true as well for dissolving one. If we could just reach into Jack's brain and wipe away his map of addiction half his battle would be won for him. Unfortunately, it is not that easy. It takes time to wire in a map and as with Susan, takes time to get rid of one. The first and most important step is as the brain is an efficient machine and does not waste space, it will speed up the rewiring process by not firing the old map you want to get rid of. The sooner the brain discovers that the map does not fit the territory the faster it will get rid of it. Therefore the first step in getting rid of an unwanted map is to stop reinforcing it. If you want to quit smoking, the more time you can go without the better, obviously! Susan kept pulling out Bills picture and sleeping with it held tightly to her chest. She also kept phoning his voicemail and listening to his greeting, just to hear his voice. This momentarily fired her neuromap and kept her from moving on as the map was reinforced. The slogan neuroscientists use to describe this process of neuroplasticity is that "neurons that fire together, wire together."

The more often two things go together, the faster they will become wired together. Conversely cells that "fire apart, wire apart." For Susan, she needs to have those experiences she had with Bill, without him. Take the dog for a walk, talk on the phone to someone else, and get rid of his matching track suit or wear it herself. By communicating to our brain that this space is being wasted it will speed up the change process. Time without firing the map allows our efficient brain to dissolves the wiring making space for new connections and new maps. Finally, install a new map as soon as possible. Do not wait for the space to get used with something else. Build a new connection.

If Victoria turned to alcohol every time she was angry. She would wire in that anger and alcohol go together. The same goes for Jack. If he used every time he had an emotional response or difficult feeling, then his map would associate drug use with those emotions. This enhances the complexity of the brain map. Victoria and Jack need to have those emotions, but do something differently like take a walk, talk to someone supportive, or exercise. Over time this will get wired in and that intense emotion will be associated with exercise, or walking.

Maps and Therapy

When people go through traumatic experience they want to be released of the negative feelings around it. There is a fine line that as professionals we must be sure not to cross between helping people "resolve the past," and letting go of the emotions surrounding a traumatic event. This is where counseling can be dangerous if it crosses the line and reinforces the pain and fear someone is holding on to. Endlessly attempting to resolve the past sets people up to relive it over and over again without getting past it. You do not want to reinforce the victim wiring.

People with traumatic experience need to take control of this by first creating a sense of safety, then learning the skills that allow them to control the bodily reaction and emotions. If a person cannot do this before any past work is attempted they are being set up for a difficult time. When a person starts with a foundation of safety and an ability to reduce their emotional response by calming the reptile and controlling the mammalian brain then it is safe to begin past focused therapy. However, not in the traditional way as the reality is the past will never be resolved and forgotten. It is more like having a virus in your computer that you can't get rid of without completely wiping out all the memory and files on the hard drive. However, you can quarantine the virus and file it away. If you open the file it will be there but the symptoms of the virus will be reduced or completely gone. Our amygdala keeps us safe by never letting go of the past, especially traumatic experience. We may have a basic emotional reaction on the mammalian level to the trauma, but we can stop the physiological over-arousal and take control of how we process the event. When the amygdala fires the fear response we have a basic emotional reaction, but it is up to us to reinforce the reaction from the neocortex, or to mitigate that reaction by reducing the reptilian and mammalian response and lead from the top part of the brain. It is the return communication of fear from the top part of the brain that enhances the fear response often causing the person to spiral. We can control this response if we choose.

Therapy and dissolving the traumatic events map will help to reduce the fear but the event will never be fully forgotten as it is there to protect you. You can dissolve the map in the neocortex though, and you do this by getting time away without firing the map telling the brain that the map no longer fits the territory and installing a new map which produces the feelings of safety and security.

Counseling can help to reorganize the information and file it away like the quarantined virus, but it cannot get the amygdala to forget or resolve it. But it is our choice to operate from the amygdala, or the neocortex. There is a time and place for most therapies, but it is important to be conscious of whether we are coming to an understanding of the past, reinforcing the negative emotions and bringing them into the present. We have to differentiate between healthy complaining to create pain to necessitate change versus reinforcing the old wiring to stay stuck and remain as the victim.

Installing a New Map

So if we know how to dissolve and rewire a map, we conversely know how to install a new map. We do this through, repetition, repetition, repetition! What does it mean to you to be able to rewire yourself? It opens the door to endless possibilities as we can change anything. The purpose of installing a new map is to create healthy behavior patterns that lead you in the direction you want to go. Use the efficiency of your unconscious mind to your advantage. "Neurons that fire together, wire together."

Secondary Emotions

Housed in our neocortex are our secondary emotions. These stem from our basic emotions and are complex as thought is added to them. For example, the emotion of shame cannot be felt without thought. Required is your projection into someone else's mind to be able to feel shame. When you feel bad about something you have done, that is guilt. To feel shame you must take your guilt and consider what determination others are making about you in their minds, otherwise shame cannot exist. So my question for you is does this serve you? Why would you choose to operate yourself this way? Basic emotion happens as a reflex and secondary emotions require thought. Therefore we can choose what emotional state we want to be in. We can create a recipe to feel however we want. We cannot directly change our feelings, but we can by changing either how we are thinking or what we are doing. This changes feelings.

Picture yourself walking down the street, the sky is blue and the sun is shining down on your face. It is warm and bright but not uncomfortable. You are smiling and happy. How do you feel? Now picture yourself in a park, huddling under a tree while a storm is blowing cold rain and wind up against you. You are shivering and cold. Now how do you feel?

We can choose our emotional state at any time. Remember

that emotions are warning signs telling you if you are on or off track. You are in control of them. Many people are led around by their emotions, misunderstanding their purpose. It is up to you to take charge of these emotions if you want to be in complete control of the direction of your life.

The more we experience an emotion the more we sensitize our self to having that emotion. Our brain develops specific receptor sites that adjust toward the repeated emotion binding more readily to the peptides of that emotion. Like dumping a certain combination of spices into a pasta sauce, peptide combinations create specific emotions. Over time of feeling the same emotion repeatedly, our brains receptor sites adjust to more efficiently process that emotion and you could even say they look for that emotion, peptide combination. More receptor sites develop for that emotion in the brain. Our receptors begin to crave the peptides and essentially our brain starts to look for that emotion. Eventually some cells will become over sensitive to this message and shut down, effectively numbing itself from that message much like a drug and alcohol dependent person becomes tolerant to their drug of choice. Other cells malfunction and die due to over stimulation of the peptide. We are wiring our self to repeat the same emotional state over and over again. We need to be conscious of how much of certain emotions we are feeding ourselves and choose what we want our overall state to be.

Our basic emotions are reflexes that come from the mammalian brain, we have them automatically, and they are limited to a few different types, it is our secondary emotions that we can control and perpetuate. These come from the higher brain functioning of the neocortex that we can control. They mix with the basic emotions and communicate back and forth.

Basic Emotions:	Anger (aggression)
	Sadness (submission)
	Fear (fright or surprise)
	Joy (acceptance, bonding, or happiness)
Additional:	Surprise
	Contempt
	Disgust
Secondary Emotions	Mixes primary emotions
	Embarrassment
	Jealousy
	Guilt
	Envy
	Pride
	Trust
	Shame, etc.

Beliefs Determine Our Outcome

We may react to any given situation with an initial basic emotional response but it is up to the thoughts we put in our head to continue with that reflex emotion, or to change it. A lot of times this is based on our beliefs. Our beliefs determine our outcome. If you believe that you can do something, you will do it. If you believe that something is impossible then you are limited by those thoughts. Beliefs enhance the thoughts we think about our self and the world. We have a decision to run off the beliefs that we learned as we were growing up, or take the opportunity to define life by installing a set of beliefs that can expand horizons and enhance life.

At your core do you believe that people are generally good and the world is safe? Or do you believe that people are out to get you, and that the world is a dark and scary place where you must protect yourself at all times. Two people with these opposite belief systems live in the same world, but would have significantly different experiences of life. The neocortex is the control panel of how we function overall. Our beliefs can tint this operation, either with fear and in effect give power to our lower level survival, and fear mechanisms, or with love, gratitude, or appreciation, giving a whole different life experience. How are you currently approaching life with fear, or joy? How you answer this will give you an indication of the type of beliefs you are currently operating from. Take a moment and decide if your beliefs are congruent with the way you want to ideally approach life. Perhaps it's time to install a new way of thinking and have a different experience of life.

A second indication of your belief system is by becoming aware of your thoughts. How do you treat yourself in your head? Do you undermine and devalue yourself? Or do you treat yourself with love and respect? Our thoughts create our reality and if your dominate level of thinking is coming from the fear center in the mammalian brain you are setting yourself up for a difficult limited life. Use your higher brain functions and treat yourself how you would treat someone that you care about. I have witnessed many people have dramatic life changing experiences by simply changing how they talk to themselves. If your neocortex is the control panel of your functioning, and you are allowing undermining thoughts about yourself to occur then you are actively limiting your life. If installing positive, loving thoughts of yourself, the world you live in will eventually evolve and reflect this new way of thinking.

After Jack learned about his map of addiction and began to cease reinforcing it with continued use, he started to install positive thoughts about himself. When he began to treat himself with respect and focus not on his past mistakes, but the opportunity that was available in his life in the moment that was before him. He went through a dramatic shift, where his concentration was not focused on the absence of using, but on what he wanted his life to be like. A lot of people stumble with this, they go to groups, attend counseling, and talk to supportive family and friends, but unfortunately when you are sitting around talking about not using, you are still talking about using, and keeping the drug front and center in your mind, making it more difficult to move on from it. Successful change comes from focusing and acting on moving forward in your life. Jack decided he wanted to go back to school to become a computer technologist. He began reading books in his field, taking on new computer challenges and made some new friends who had similar interests without the history of drug use. He followed their recipe of how to live a life without substance using and before he knew it, months went by without a relapse. Last time I saw him he was well on his way to a completely different life. His internal self-talk reflected a person who felt good about himself and the world.

Positive affirmations can become wired in beliefs that work to drive your life in a positive direction. It is always better to use process statements as affirmations as they are more believable than sweeping grandiose statements. Making declarations like "I'm the funniest person alive, or fittest or fastest" undermine the affirmation as your brain can easily find information that questions these statements. As soon as you use global accusations that on one level your brain knows that it is not entirely true or can question, then you are less likely to accept the statement and therefore undermines the affirmation. Instead say "I'm getting stronger everyday, or faster, or fitter, leaner, healthier, smarter etc." These are process affirmations that will not be undermined by information of the contrary. Unless of course your name is Usain Bolt, do not say you are the fastest person alive, say "I'm becoming faster everyday."

Briefcase Tools for Operating the Neocortex

- Dissolve old neuromaps by letting time pass without reinforcing them

- Create new maps through repetition that move you in the direction you want to go

- Take control of your beliefs, and secondary emotions to create a recipe for success

- Install some life supporting new beliefs and positive affirmations

Chapter 6

Operating Yourself for Maximum Performance

"You must have control of the authorship of your own destiny. The pen that writes your life story must be held in your own hand."

Irene C. Kassorla

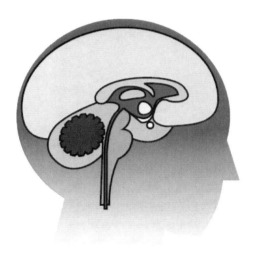

Up to this point the purpose of the materials covered in this book is to lay the foundation of knowledge necessary to take control of how you operate yourself. For those who have read the information the following will be a quick review, but for those who skipped right to this chapter, it will give you a hangnail sketch of the brain and how it operates, leading you to actively putting this knowledge into action to optimize your functioning.

Overview Sketch of the Brain

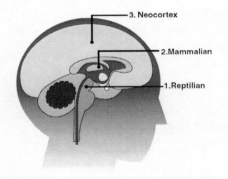

Basically we have three brains in one; the reptilian, mammalian, and neocortex.

These three brains are inter-connected, yet responsible for separate tasks. They developed in order of 'survival need.' First, the reptilian emerged to keep us safe from external threats; then came the mammalian brain to protect us from internal threats; finally, the neocortex developed to give us advanced community, cooperation, and intelligence as we aren't physically as strong as most members of the reptile and mammal community. Difficulties often arise when we function solely out of the survival skills of reptilian or the "fear warehouse" of mammalian brain. On the other hand, the neocortex houses our ability for cost-benefit analysis, foresight, goal setting, logic, rational thinking, empathy, and abstract thinking. Most important of all though, is that this is where our control panel of all our functioning is. With this comes the opportunity to take control of even our most basic unconscious survival mechanisms housed in the reptilian brain. This is where we choose how to operate ourselves.

Now that we have completed the review, it's important to understand our fear circuitry and how to break the fear loop to pave the way to optimize your functioning and create your own success plan.

The Fear Circuitry

The neuromap, which was described earlier, is the key to proactively changing how we operate our self and decreasing our fear response. We can wire in a pattern of thoughts that triggers our fear circuitry, tuning in our mammalian brain and survival mechanisms to activate the sympathetic nervous system response. This mobilizes our reptilian brain to release cortisol and adrenaline into the blood steam gearing us up for action. The problem is that most modern threats are abstract. They're not concrete like a tiger chasing you down the street. They are abstract like money issues, emails, phone calls and other things that we really have to think about. However, our survival system responds the same way to abstract stimulus as it does to concrete. That is why we can think our self into a panic attack.

To solve this problem we need to wire in a pattern of thoughts that puts us in a state that optimizes performance. Affirmations help to do this by pairing the positive thoughts and associated feelings of the affirmation with our belief around our self-identity or our perception of the world. Once this is wired in we then associate the positive thought to our reality and the two become linked. The positive thought that is wired in does not trigger the fear circuitry rather it triggers a parasympathetic response that turns on the calming, growth and development system. As a result the blood flows to the top part of the brain and we think clearer, make better decisions, and have a positive perception of the world. Having an ingrained positive neuromap sets you up to live a better life versus living in the fear response that is cyclical, as fear triggers more fear. Below the following example of you and the tiger is a visual representation of the fear response loop.

You Versus the Tiger

You are downtown and walk around a corner and to your surprise, a tiger is standing in the middle of the street looking at you with wanting eyes. It looks hungry, angry, and has that certain gleam in his eye that tells you he perceives you as a giant pork chop.

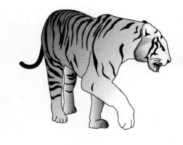

Immediately, your senses filter out all other information, focussing on nothing else but the tiger. Thoughts of unpaid bills, picking up milk on the way home, and your family values vanish, only you and the tiger exist at this moment in time. At least that is what your brain is saying.

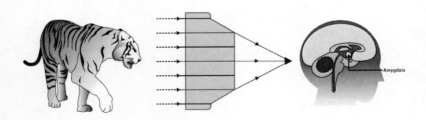

The sensory information of the tiger is passed through the filter right to your amygdala in the mammalian brain where the determination of safety is made. The amygdala makes this decision based on past information or prior experience, but in this case, it doesn't take long to decide that your safety is at risk and therefore your fear circuitry is activated. In another circumstance such as if you were at a zoo, the representation of the tiger most likely in a cage may allow your amygdala to decide that you are safe and instead of holding onto the information, the amygdala passes it onto the neocortex for further processing. However, when your safety is at risk the amygdala cuts the neocortex out of the loop, as you cannot waste your time thinking when you need to act. The amygdala decides that the fear response is needed to keep you safe and tells the reptilian brain to fire up the survival mechanisms. Your heart rate and blood pressure increase as your body releases cortisol and adrenaline into the blood stream, as these chemicals increase your strength and speed. Digestion shuts down as the blood flows to the muscles to mobilize them for action. In the brain, blood flow to the neocortex is decreased and redirected to the reptilian and mammalian brains. There is no need for logic, reason or creativity when you are running for your life.

After the sympathetic, activating response comes the immediate action of either, fight, flight, or freeze. In this case, freeze is not going to work as the tiger is already looking at you like you are a giant pork chop and its next meal. Fight is not going to work because you have nothing to use as a weapon, and quite honestly my money is on the tiger. The tiger is far enough away so you turn and run back around the corner, into a store, and hide safely in the bathroom.

The safety question is then returned back to your senses to scan the environment. The new information set is filtered and brought to your amygdala, which now decides that you are safe, and directs the information to your neocortex for more complex processing. This is where you start to question, "hmm, a tiger downtown, that's weird." Later you see on the news that a tiger escaped form the zoo and then everything makes sense. Now that your neocortex is involved you can analyze the situation, what you did, and how to handle it in the future. You could also install some regrets, shame, or feelings of guilt if you really wanted to, but in this situation as in most, it is unhelpful and unnecessary.

Fear Response Loop

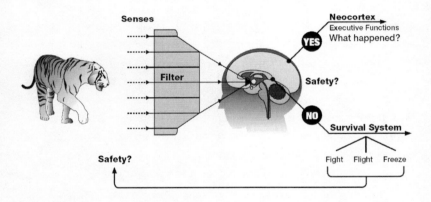

Survival and Today's Society

The problem is that today our society is safe. We don't have tigers or other predators running through our streets, but our survival mechanisms get turned on the same way from abstract stressors, or our thoughts, as from concrete stimuli such as a tiger. Now as I sit in this chair writing this book, my phone is ringing, emails are coming in, and my awareness gets heightened the same way it would if there was a concrete threat. My survival mechanisms, on the reptilian level have no thought, and on the mammalian level have no logic, and react as if the phone ringing was a tiger posturing.

Our thoughts have the biggest impact in this reaction as we can consciously choose to turn off our fear circuitry, or we can contribute to the cycle of fear. We contribute to the cycle of fear by instead of analyzing the situation, understanding it, and filing it away, we relive it, over and over again. Often it becomes a story about how unsafe the world is. The repetition of this story causes it to become wired into your perception of the world and from that perception, real or not, you operate yourself.

When a fear state is maintained, your body remains in an activated state and over time it begins to wear down as the stress hormones wreak havoc while running through your blood stream. In due course, the high arousal state depletes your body of its nutrient and their reserves, which causes the body to breakdown. It's like trying to avoid paying off a loan shark, eventually he's going to catch up with you and snap off a digit. Without time in the calming system, to grow and repair itself, your body becomes tired, lethargic, depressed, and anxious.

It is of vital importance that you make sure you spend more time in growth, than in activation. The growth state will reduce the cortisol and adrenaline released in the blood stream and will give your body the nutrients it needs to repair itself and to replenish its reserves. This will decrease tiredness, lethargy, depression, anxiety, and other body responses to stress. Wiring in a belief system and positive neuromap which keeps you in the calming system will also allow you to create a healthier, happier, bigger life.

Changes That Maximize Effectiveness

To make changes and operate your self with maximum effectiveness it takes more than just thinking the right thoughts, or feeling positive emotions, it takes action. All the happy thoughts and feelings in the world will not help you make any real change if it is not accompanied by massive action. Lack of consistent action is where counselling can fail. You can leave my office feeling like the king of the world, but if you do nothing to build on that state, you will inevitably return the next week feeling the way you did before you came to me in the first place. The necessary ingredient to change is action and true change happens in between sessions, not within the session.

Spectrum of Action

Perhaps the greatest failure in counseling is that sometimes counselors encourage people to express their thoughts and feelings, without creating momentum or a plan for change. Back to the rosebush, it may help you to change your perception of living in a thorn bush, reframing it as living in a rosebush, but too often that is as far as it goes. You feel better about your situation but never make any real changes. Real change comes from the action you take. It comes from changing what you have been doing and installing some new actions that will change your circumstance. Action will allow you to get up and out of the thorns and live free.

All Talk - No Action

Action is on a spectrum where at one end there is all talk or thought and no action and on the other is all action, without thought. All talk no action is where counseling can make problems worse. There is a benefit to expressing and emoting as the participant feels better and maybe even accomplished without ever actually doing anything. However, with all thought and no action, we tend to over think things and change appears more difficult than it needs to be. We procrastinate, often opening ourselves up to being more sensitive, scared, fearful, which decreases our energy. Sometimes in this state we experience a complete absence of anger, which, believe it or not, is a problem.

Anger is a powerful force, when used correctly it can help us get things done, increase motivation, and give us strength. Obviously, it can cause us some significant problems as well, as we are more prone to make mistakes when we are angry. Mistakes occur when the blood is flowing to that middle and lower parts of the brain, mobilizing our body for action, and not to our neocortex. Since the logical center is not being activated we are not thinking things through and using our executive functions to prevent mistakes. Unless we consciously take control with the neocortex, to use the anger to our advantage, we are opening ourselves to making mistakes in the moment.

All Action - No Thought

The other end of the spectrum is all action, with no thought. Here anger can be a great motivator as we act with boldness, often impulsively, and because we're not activating the human part of the brain, we act with high energy and strength. We don't take the time to over think things and thus don't allow our thoughts to undermine our actions. The problem on this side is that due to the impulsivity of action and no thought, we often make poor choices in the moment. All action and not thought is where the drug addict lives in when they are in a craving state.

To operate effectively we must bridge this gap between the two extremes and work somewhere in the middle. This space is the efficiency zone and where we get things done, using our human capabilities of thought and action. Here we don't allow the fear that over thinking creates to undermine us, and we don't take impulsive action either. The efficiency zone is where goal setting takes place. It's the zone where we don't procrastinate, or let our thoughts throw us into a state of overwhelm.

Combating Overwhelm

Overwhelm comes from one, two, or both conditions of either doing too much, or having too much to do. If we are doing too much, it's time to take a healthy break and relax. If it's having too much to do, then we need to stop procrastinating, break the tasks down into manageable goals, and take action. In the efficiency zone, you will be surprised how much can be accomplished. Life is a series of sprint and recovery zones. Equally important to working hard, is resting and rebuilding yourself so you are ready for the next sprint. Make sure you counter time spent in activation with more time in growth that will help you repair yourself.

Rockslide Momentum

As an addictions counselor the one thing that most amazes me is that when people start working in a healthy direction it's incredible how fast things start to come together. Knowing that taking on too much often creates a recipe for failure, or the state of overwhelm, that often leads to failure, it's important to focus on the little things within their circle of control. By focusing on what a person can do currently to change, they start building momentum. I often use the rockslide analogy for my clients. I tell them to focus first on getting some pebbles to move. Rock slides begin as a few small pebbles start to roll down and bump into a few other pebbles then those pebbles bump into more and more until the group of little pebbles have enough force and momentum to crash into bigger rocks, causing them to slide down the hill. Together they smash into other rocks and before you know it the whole mountainside is coming crashing down. I have seen this concept of building momentum work in peoples lives countless times. People often question if this can truly happen, but it inevitably does. This doesn't mean there won't be any hidden hurdles that present themselves, but it does mean that once the momentum is going in the right direction the obstacles are moved out of the way or surmounted. It's our inner obstacles that we need to pay attention to for they have the power to slow us down or even stop us if we let them.

Environments That Don't Support Us

We create environments that support how we treat ourselves. Thinking poorly and talking negatively about ourselves wears us out and drains our energy. The thoughts we think are related to how we feel and behave. When we feel badly we often react by drinking too much alcohol, or eating junk food or overeating. Emotionally eating is a huge problem in North America.

The survival function that developed as the neocortex evolved can't tell the different between a thought and what is real. So when you think negative thoughts about yourself the brain perceives this information as a threat, which causes your survival mechanisms to become active. In the case of emotional eating, the brain believes your survival is at risk and clicks into craving so that you will act on the threat of scarcity, even though the threat isn't real. So eating fatty foods does two things, puts on some weight so you can make it through those winter months, and secondly releases dopamine in your reward system, which feels good, elevating mood. However, you continue to talk poorly to yourself and then feel guilt for eating poorly, or drinking too much, leading to more negative thoughts, feelings, and behaviors and eventually your environment will reflect this. You may isolate yourself, spend hours watching TV. Even if you do go out and meet people, you find the ones that will treat you poorly, or drink too much alcohol or use drugs. This cycle will continue until you decide to change. Once you do it's amazing how soon you can stop the old undermining thoughts and wire in a new pattern that makes you healthier, happier, and strong.

Creating Environments That Support Us

Changing how you talk to yourself changes how you feel about yourself, and this alters what you do, and how you behave. This chain of events can shift the circumstance of your life and the environment you create, and before you know it you start to meet people who treat you with respect. This all starts with breaking habitual negative thoughts. Over a short period of time your new way of thinking and being gets wired into your brain. I have noticed that thinking differently becomes so natural to people that they forget that they used to talk to themselves negatively. I've heard people say that they can't believe how cruel they used to be to themselves. To create change we must consciously take control and operate ourselves from the higher brain functions of our neocortex. It's easy to do, but most of us are unaware of how to do it and that is why I wrote this book.

The C-Force and Momentum

A decade ago, I was working for a group home and needed to get my class four driver's license so that I would be able to transport kids around in the van. In the driver information book, it discussed centrifugal force. This is the gravitational force that is created by forward momentum. When you slow down or turn the C-force is the gravitational pressure that pushes you to continue the way you were travelling before. If you apply this same principle to life, it really makes sense. It is not just our forward momentum that pushes us to continue on the path we were heading, but our living systems, such as family, environment, career, physical condition, emotional being, etc. When there is a change in any part of a system, it forces change on the rest of the system.

How this applies to people is that most people don't like forced change and when you change, it naturally causes change in others' lives, so they consciously or not, pressure you to stay in the place you have always been, and do exactly what is expected, what they are familiar with. They hold the expectation that you will maintain your place in the system and not cause any ripples. When you are making a life change, even the people who outwardly support you, sometimes unconsciously work to undermine you.

The C-force of your life propels you to continue on the path you were always on. So when making a life change you, not only have to work to create the changes you are seeking, but need to stay mindful of the C-force that pulls you away from success. Even a small change, such as internally changing how you operate yourself draws the C-force in. Take the following husband and wife for example.

Constance and Lee and the C-force

Constance is unhappy about her weight and attempts to diet. Her husband Lee would like her thinner, and knows that she would benefit from feeling healthier, more confident, attractive and possibly even happier. They both would gain by this change. Constance immediately makes some changes, throws out junk food, becomes more active, begins a diet, and starts to change the momentum of her life. Then the C-force kicks in. Lee takes her out to dinner and then goes grocery shopping and buys the junk food that she had previously loved. He is not consciously trying to undermine her, but his actions seek to keep her in the same place, doing the same things she has always done. A fight ensues as she is not feeling supported. She accuses him of purposely undermining her, then breaks down and emotionally eats the junk food that Lee had so kindly purchased. Constance throws in the towel, quits her diet, possibly blaming him, and feels worse than before about herself. She resumes her place in the family system and Lee as he historically has done takes her out to dinner, or buys her a treat to "make her feel better." The cycle continues.

Change was forced on Lee by Constance changing her activity level, and altering their eating habits. What would have helped set her up for success? Constance could have helped Lee get on board with the healthier living plan, and overhauled the whole system. Or she could have slowed down the changes and decrease the C-force. She also could have pulled her self out of the system, or leave the system for a short time while she established new habits which may have created success for her. However, leaving for a time is often not that effective.

It's like sending a drug addict to rehab only to return to their life exactly how they left it. It's only a matter of time before the C-force pulls the person back into place. Often it happens within the first couple of days of their return from treatment.

The C-Force Working for You

It is not only your environmental system that can contribute to making change more difficult. When you make any turn in life the C-force pulls you in your previous direction. Maintaining the changes over time creates sustained change which draws this force back in harnessing its power to work for you. When this happens often things begin to fit together as things start to fall in place. As you approach life with the C-force on your side, you continue to build on your new momentum and massive change becomes easier. All because you got up out of the thorn bush and took mindful action towards creating a new life.

Chris Douglas

Chapter 7

Your Personalized Success Plan

"Man's mind, once stretched by a new idea,
never regains its original dimensions."

Oliver Wendell Holmes, Jr.

Your Personalized Success Plan

The following section is about maximizing your functioning. It's about moving your life forward and giving yourself a bigger, happier, healthier, better life.

Chris Douglas

Trouble Shooting Guide Introduction

Directly following this section is a troubleshooting guide for people
who are dealing with anxiety, depression, anger, and more. In that
section you will learn to put the information from this book into
practice in order to deal with impairments to your functioning.
When people are struggling with issues like anxiety it can hold
them back and keep them crippled with fear to the point that all
they want to do is hide under their bed sheets. They become so
fearful that they draw everything in and their life becomes small as
all that is real to them is their need to survive. If you have issue with
fear, anxiety, depression or alcohol or drug abuse, check out the
Trouble Shooting Guide. You have an opportunity to push the
boundaries of your life and make it bigger. The choice is yours.

Future Reflection Questions

First you must decide what you want out of life. Where do you
want to be in one, two, five or twenty years? How do you want to
feel as you travel through life? What kind of person do you want to
be? What kind of beliefs do you want to have? What level of energy
do you want to approach life with? Is there a part of your
personality, or feelings about your self that you are not 100% happy
with and would like to change?

As you think about these questions take a sheet of paper out
and begin brainstorming. Don't judge or criticizes yourself because
at this stage you just want to write without limiting yourself.
Sometimes just getting the momentum of the pen moving is
enough to draw out what you truly want out of life.

Past Reflection Questions

Project yourself into the future looking back, what are you most proud of? Who are you surrounded by? What do you appreciate about the way you lived your life? Keep writing.

Are there any experiences you have had that make you beam with excitement? Write those down.

Future Reference Points

Now, as clearly as you can create a picture of your life at some point or many points in the future such as 1, 2, 5, 10, or 20 years. The clearer you can define this the easier the next part is.

Steps to Move You Towards Your Desired Future

Next, write down 5 or 10 steps that you need to do to make that picture a reality. What is the first step? What can you do right now to bring yourself closer to achieving that picture of a perfect life for you? What can you do tonight, tomorrow and this week? How good are you going to feel when you have these steps completed? How good are you going to feel when you make this perfect life a reality? Put yourself in that state. What thoughts will you be thinking and how will you talk to yourself? What actions will you take? What feelings are you feeling? Feel this right now. As you envision this future, what does it feel like in your body? Try to get a body sense because it makes the picture more real. Remember that the brain can't tell the difference between thoughts and imagination.

Make a list of the possible roadblocks that may slow your progress. How will you deal with these?

What energy zone are you going to need to be in? Red, yellow, or green. What type of food helps put you in that energy zone? Red, yellow or, green. What is an example of a few green foods?

What is the pain you will experience if you do not make this picture a reality? What will you lose? How is your life limited or confined by not taking the necessary steps to give yourself a great life? Feel this pain, make it real, and ask yourself what pleasure you will experience by making this picture a reality.

How are you going to talk to yourself to empower yourself to stay on track and make this picture a reality?

What habits do you need to break to move closer to your new life? What habits or neuromaps do you need to install? How are you going to operate yourself now that you have the knowledge necessary to control your functioning and maximize your capabilities? What actions are you going to take right now?

Put your pen down and go do it, because you want the power of positive momentum working for you if you are going to make this change a reality.

What's in Your Briefcase?

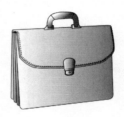

Briefcase Tools for Operating the Human Reptile

- Deep Breathe to manage the activating survival response

- Manage your state through posture control

- Tune into your fuel and energy systems

- Be your own expert and examine the relationship between food and energy

- To change your physical health you must change your communication through sending a different message of your lifestyle through fuel and movement

- To enhance processing of food take ten deep breaths before you eat to put yourself in a relaxing state to optimize digestion

Briefcase Tools for Operating Your Inner Mammal

- Deep breathe to calm the reptile

- Put yourself in a state of gratitude, appreciation, or love.

- Give yourself breaks to reset the filter

- Spend more time in the calming growth system then in protection

- Eat in a growth state

- Send positive thoughts to your filter to perceive the world in a positive light

- Motivate yourself with the pain and pleasure principle

- Use your emotional guidance system to know if you are on track

Briefcase Tools for Operating the Neocortex

- Dissolve old neuromaps by letting time pass without reinforcing them

- Create new maps that move you in the direction you want to go

- Take control of your beliefs, and secondary emotions to create a recipe for success

- Install some life supporting new beliefs and positive affirmations

Appendix

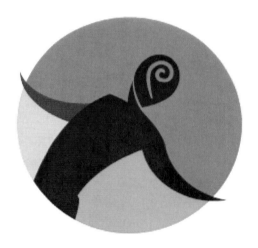

Troubleshooting Guide

Operating Yourself with Alcohol and/or Drug Dependency

Some common questions regarding substance dependence:

My forty two year old son Jimmy, steals from me, lies, and is belligerent towards his father and me when he is using and after he has relapsed. He wasn't raised like this. Why is he doing this?

You must understand that if Jimmy is addicted to a substance than he is operating himself from a different place than you or I. Family values are ingrained in the neocortex. When someone becomes drug or alcohol dependent it's like they start working from the mammalian and reptilian part of the brain. In the mammalian brain we have basic emotion, motivation and memory, but there is no logic. That is a higher brain function that does not exist at this level. The more substance dependent a person becomes the less and less they are using their higher brain functions and the more they are operating from the mammalian brain and running off the pain from withdrawal and/or cravings. At the mammalian level this intense pain can feel life threatening as the need to use is perceived as necessary for survival. Does a coyote stop to think about his family values before he attacks a neighborhood cat? Or would a snake consider a mouse's feelings before swallowing him whole? Of course not, the good news is that your son is still human and can relearn to override these intense cravings by managing his reptilian and mammalian brain with his neocortex.

Why do people get cravings?

This is not just related to substance abuse but is a normal process. We can get cravings for food like sugar and fat but that is a little different process. There is a historical biological reason for our sugar and fat cravings as in hunter gatherer societies early humans out in the forest knew if a berry was safe to eat by tasting it. Sweet taste meant that it was okay to eat, while bitter was a signal that it is poisonous. As for fat, we crave it as it is the most nutrient dense food and is essential to survival as it is not only used as a fuel source, but is important to brain functioning and healthy cell functioning.

Substance cravings come from physical withdrawal or change. As we have a change in behavior it is new and uncomfortable. Our brain wants to follow the old pattern even if it is unhealthy because it is what is known. Cravings emerge to pressure us to follow the old pattern even if it is unhealthy, and reinforce the old behavior. We need to continue to change the behavior and do something different to deal with the trigger. The craving may increase in the short term as the brain fights harder to make you follow the old pattern. Over time cravings subside as the brain dissolves old wired in behavior pattern and installs a new pattern. The new behavior is reinforced through use. Eventually triggers lead to new behavior without thought process involved. Cravings are no longer needed and brain is rewired.

Why do people get depressed when quitting drugs and alcohol?

There is a passageway in the brain called the dopamine reward passageway and a part of it is situated in the nucleus accumbens. This is the brain's reward center, which is in the mammalian brain. When we use drugs or alcohol this is the part that gives us that good feeling of reward. Remember that within the mammalian brain lays our motivation, memory and reward center and has no capacity for logic as it develops to approximately age two. This causes problems as what we want most is to move towards pleasure and avoid pain. Drugs and alcohol immediately do this and work on the reward center which is situated right next to our memory center. So it makes sense from a brain stand point why people become addicted to substances as our memory and pleasure systems work closely together without needing to engage the logic of the neocortex.

It is only when the pain of using starts to outweigh the pleasure that people start to realize that they may be addicted and that it is becoming a serious problem. Often they lose work, relationships, and find themselves up on charges because of their use and they decide it is time to quit. In the nucleus accumbens prolonged drug and alcohol use causes the release of the neurotransmitter dopamine. If we blow up a section of the reward center we can see that dopamine travels down to the edge of a cell in a vesicle that works much like a balloon filled with water. When it gets to the edge it releases the dopamine into the gap or synaptic cleft where it accumulates and binds to the receptor sites on the next cell. When this transaction is completed the result is a good feeling or the "high." Over time the brain and body, who work towards homeostasis, or keeping things "the same," start to realize that it is feeling too much pleasure that it has not earned. This artificial reward builds up and the body takes steps to make things normal again. It does this by reducing the number of receptor sites available to receive the dopamine. This process is called down regulation.

Dopamine Reward System

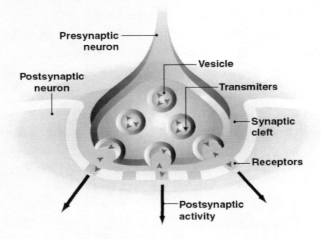

If I drink a six pack of beer a day for four months, the first day I may be intoxicated and feeling good, but as days go by the alcohol will not hit me as hard, and by the fourth month, I may not be feeling the effects at all. This is because of down regulation and is the reason we get tolerance.

The beer is no longer giving me as much pleasure so I either increase my use, or in this case, I decide to quit drinking. A few weeks go by without any alcohol and I am struggling because I am doing things that normally would give me a natural reward, however it's not feeling as good as it should. This is because the receptor sites are still deconstructed to accommodate the prior artificial dopamine release. This problem is known as anhedonia or the feeling of an absence of pleasure and is a major contributor to depression. Time passes without the artificial release and the homeostatic response kicks in again as the brain realizes that you are doing natural things that should feel good, but are not getting the pleasure from it. So the body responds by reconstructing some new receptor sites, a process known as up regulation. If you decide to go back to drinking a six pack a day again, this process will happen again a lot quicker as there are some memory effects in this process.

Research into the reward center of rats indicates that there is a significant increase of dopamine in the gap between cells depending on what activity the rats are engaged in. Rat brain function is similar to humans and the approximate percentage increase of dopamine is found during the following activities:

Nicotine	225%
Alcohol	180%
Morphine	200%
Cocaine	350%
Methamphetamine	1200%

Compare this to the natural rewards of:

Food	150%
Sex	200%

Drugs and alcohol also affect other parts of the body. For example opiates work on the pain system numbing the pain response. Other neurotransmitters are also involved but this is here to illustrate what happens on the dopamine system as it is a key part of addiction. People who become addicted to gambling, sex, and/or eating do so because of the dopamine response.

To enhance up regulation it is important to give the body time away from artificially stimulating the dopamine reward system. Second, stimulate the reward system as much as possible through natural means such as eating, or having sex. In addition you want to give the body proper nutrients necessary to rebuild the depleted neurotransmitters. There are two important amino acids or proteins essential to neurotransmitter development: tryptophan and tyrosine. Tryptophan is found in meat, poultry, tofu, and seafood. Tyrosine is found in bananas, milk, sunflower seeds, and turkey. It's important to give the body the building blocks necessary to facilitate this change process. It may take time and differs between individuals depending on genetics, nutrition, stress level, how much each drug was used, and for how long, but you're your body will recover.

What types of triggers are there and how do I manage them?

Triggers can be anything, the most common are people, places, things, time of the day, emotional states, feelings, cups, anxiety, depression, embarrassment, fear, anything that is processed through the senses, memories etc. I once worked with a young man who every time he had a shower he would feel triggered and he could not figure out why as when he was abusing cocaine he barely showered at all! The problem was that cocaine increases the heart rate which raises the body's temperature. When he cleaned up and took a hot shower in the morning the heat from the shower would cause his body temperature to rise and before he knew it he was in a craving state. Just having the knowledge of this was enough for him to take control. He knew he had to shower a lot of times without using cocaine and installed some coping strategies before, during and after his shower to help him manage this. He deep breathed to calm his reptilian survival response, and focused on how appreciative he is that he was clean from cocaine use. This calmed his amygdala from firing up his survival mechanisms and put the blood flow to the top parts of the brain, thus taking control of his state. After some time of practicing his new coping strategies, he found that not only had the triggered state ceased, but every time he showered he left feeling on top of the world as he was in a complete state of appreciation and ready to have a spectacular day. This new experience around showering became a positive neuromap that he used sometimes if he was having a bad day. He would take a shower and restart the day in a completely different state.

How do you quit using?

It is different for everyone, but it starts with managing your state. Calming the reptile and putting your self in an appreciative state. It is essential to make sure you are dealing with things from the neocortex and not letting the pain of withdrawal or an emotional moment pull you down into operating from the mammalian brain or worse. You are in charge, and you must stay in charge and operate from your neocortex.

Operating Yourself with Anxiety

What is the purpose of anxiety?

Anxiety is a fear response. Its function is to keep us safe however, it does so at the cost of limiting your life, if you let it get out of control. It's like having an over controlling spouse. In the short term it's easier to avoid the conflict and give in to it, but in the long term you are contributing to the problem because you are actively limiting your life.

Who gets anxiety?

Everyone experiences anxiety in one form or another. Whether it's significant life limiting anxiety, or small and manageable, everyone has had anxiety. If you don't, you might want to check your pulse because your heart has probably stopped beating.

Is anxiety normal?

Anxiety is a normal part of being human and we all experience different levels of anxiety throughout our lives depending on what we are doing, experiencing, thinking, sleeping, eating etc. Anxiety is normal, you would not get out of bed in the morning if you didn't have some anxiety, whether it is going to work to earn money to pay the bills, or getting to school to pass a test. Anxiety helps us get things done.

In the field of sport psychology, studies were conducted on high performance athletes and how they manage their anxiety during a sporting event. Their findings led them to suggest that there is a performance zone which looks like an inverted-u (see diagram below).

Low anxiety may not have negative physical consequences but is not ideal for performance. This is why if you watch athletes before competitions some may be psyching themselves up by jumping or doing pushups because they are trying to increase their arousal and bring it into their performance zone. Others may be deep breathing or listening to relaxing music while sitting alone. These athletes are prone to higher levels of anxiety and use anxiety reducing strategies to lower their arousal and move it down into their peak performance zone.

Most people fall on the right side of the graph where they have to work on reducing their anxiety instead of increasing it. The best performances occur when the individual is neither too aroused, nor under aroused.

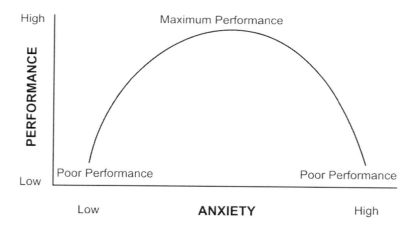

What triggers anxiety?

Anxiety can be triggered both internally and externally. First, it's important to become aware of your symptoms of when you are starting to feel anxiety as this will lead to earlier detection, which will help you deal with it sooner before it is out of control and may cause a panic attack.

There are many physical symptoms of anxiety. These may include:

> Tense muscles
> Trembling
> Churning stomach
> Nausea
> Diarrhea
> Headache
> Backache
> Heart palpitations/ increased heart rate and/or adrenaline rush
> Numbness or "pins and needles" in arms, hands or legs
> Sweating/flushing

When people are experiencing high levels of anxiety they often have specific behaviors associated with being in an anxious state.

Some of these may include:

> Pacing
> Using drugs or drinking alcohol
> Smoking
> Laying in bed
> Stuttering
> Shallow breathing
> Avoiding situations
> Restlessness

Thoughts that enhance anxiety may include:

> "I'm a loser."
> "I need to drink/use."
> "What is wrong with me?"

Anxiety increasing self talk tends to give away personal control and power as it tends to be negative, pessimistic, problem focused, permanent, and hope destroying.

How do you take control of anxiety?

Thoughts, feelings, and behaviors are connected and when one aspect is affected, all are influenced. We cannot change our feelings directly. To change our feelings we must first either change our thoughts or change our behaviors.

The basic skills taught in counseling to manage anxiety typically include:

Deep breathing
Exercise
Walk
Get plenty of rest
Talk to someone supportive
Avoid caffeine
Eat healthy food
Yoga

Changing how you communicate to yourself with your thoughts will also help you to reduce your level of anxiety. Some suggestions may include:

"I have felt anxious in the past and have made it through."
"I can do this."

Use imagery and create a relaxing scene to focus on. Learn to replace "negative self talk" with "positive self talk." Replace "I can't do this" with "I am going to feel stronger and healthier when I get through this."

Challenge negative thoughts with new empowering thoughts. Remember the connection of the new thoughts and behaviors. If you change your anxiety enhancing thoughts or behavior you will produce a different feeling state. Everybody is capable of controlling their state by using the connection between thoughts and behaviors to alter that feeling state.

The above information is the standard techniques taught in both group and individual therapy. They can be very helpful, but I would like to take them one step further and explain what is happening to our bodies and how to change this anxiety response. The following section will describe the brain's response, the fear network, the physical sensations, and what we can do to stop them, then tell a story to illustrate the points, but first I'll start with a rattlesnake story.

How do you calm the anxious reptile?

How do you calm the reptile? Deep breathe. Imagine you are hiking in the desert and hear a hiss and a rattle. You look down and there is an angry rattlesnake in front of you. You both know you're not its dinner. However, you are in its territory and it's angry. You need to calm the situation so you first deep breathe. This reduces the survival response whether it is triggered by something external such as the snake, or internal such as an ingrained irrational fear response. After you deep breathe and lower your heart rate, putting yourself into a calming state rather than activation, you back out of the situation to safety. The rattler is just posturing to keep you away from its home and doesn't chase you.

What happens physically when you get anxiety?

We have a biological fear system that is woven throughout our brain that creates a neurological fear network. This system started developing 100 million years ago with the development of the brain stem (the lowest part of our brain). The purpose of this system was and still is survival. In the brain stem our instinctual fears are held. The brain stem is also known as the reptilian brain. This is the first part of the brain to develop in the womb. The reptilian brain is incapable of higher thought and can't process emotions such as love or happiness. Again, this is why a lizard doesn't make a good pet; it is only concerned with survival and will never know its name or come when it's called.

The second area involved in the fear network is known as the mammalian brain, which is the second area to evolve. The mammalian brain is also called the limbic system which is the emotional and motivational center of the brain. Within this area lies our "warehouse of fear" called the amygdala. The amygdala is a memory center for emotion and in particular stores memories of painful and threatening experiences. The amygdala is more sophisticated than the reptilian brain as it can evaluate fears at a very basic level, however this is on a very primitive level.

The amygdala is directly connected to the body's action system, the endocrine glands which produce hormones that have many functions including protecting the body from danger. The two primary survival hormones are cortisol and adrenaline which are often referred to as the stress hormones. These hormones give us the ability to run faster, fight harder, and increase our strength. People speak of stories such as a grandmother lifting a car off her grandchild. These two hormones are what would make this possible.

The release of these hormones instigates the release of

excitatory neurotransmitters in the brain, which increase alertness and increase the psychological and physical symptoms of fear. Such as we discussed earlier-increased heart rate, high blood pressure, butterflies in the stomach, insomnia, and jitteriness reinforce the feeling of fear which increases anxiety. The point of going through all of this biology is not necessarily to learn all of these mechanisms, but to understand that these structures evolved with a purpose: survival of a species.

Millions of years ago people literally ran off their extra stress hormones. Today, we sit in our offices, staring at our computer screens and the only threat to our survival is finding out that someone switched our coffee with decaf. Actually, our only threats are threats of perception. Will we have enough money to pay our bills? What I mean by this is that money does not really exist. It's only paper that we have created some symbolic attachment to. Historically you wouldn't stop running from a dinosaur if somebody threatened you with unpaid bills, but today we have people who work in lion cages in order to make some paper to pay their bills.

We have this hardwired system for dealing with daily survival threats, but we do not face any threats. We don't move around enough to use up our extra "energy." This creates anxiety problems. When I'm sitting at my desk it does me no good to have cortisol and adrenaline build up in my system, maybe I can type faster, but there is no real survival benefit to this. Fortunately, we can control this system. Humans have a large cerebral neocortex, specifically frontal lobes which allow us to take control of this system. The neocortex which means new brain was the last structure to develop during evolution and in the womb. This is the site of the human intellect, gives us creativity, allows us to do cost benefits analysis, play the tape through and use abstract reasoning skills as well as store long term memories. The neocortex evaluates messages from the two lower brain areas and can over-rule actions of the two.

What happens to trigger our fear network?

Two things, first we can think about our anxieties as we described in the self talk section earlier, or we experience through our environmental interpretations. There is approximately 400 billion bits of information being processed per second, however we are only aware of 2000. Something happens in our environment, we filter it through our senses and the amygdala makes a snap judgment based on past experience whether there is a threat or not. If it perceives a pleasurable interaction such as a child smiling to you as you walk by, then a hormone will be released and you will reflexively smile back, then the neocortex will get involved.

If the interaction is perceived as a threat the amygdala will stimulate the fear system and the body will mobilize to fight, flight, or freeze. The stress hormones will be released to arouse the body to survive. The body will shut down digestion which may produce the symptom of butterflies in the stomach and you may feel a dry mouth. Your heart rate will increase as well as respiration and oxygenation giving the muscles more fuel to react. Other symptoms of fear (hyper arousal) may include fast breathing or panting, turning pale, dilated pupils, shivers or feeling cold, voice change, and shaky legs which can be helped by pressing feet to the floor to tighten quadriceps.

With all of these physical sensations, what can we do to stop this?

We need to use our neocortex to take control and do the following.

First, we need to deep breathe as within 5 to 10 deep breathes our body switches off the physical aspects of the fear system putting us into our calming system (parasympathetic nervous system). Second, we need to put ourselves in a state of appreciation (love, gratitude) as when we are in this state it shuts down the blood flow to the amygdala. Less blood flow means less oxygen which in turn means less fuel for the amygdala. Third, gets lots of exercise as it will allow the body to use up the rest of the hormones in the blood stream.

Can you give an example to better illustrate this?

A caveman is walking down the path to get some water. The bushes next to him rustle. His amygdala perceives a threat and he is off and running back to his cave. When he reaches his tribe they grunt asking him what is wrong. He thinks for a second and replies that there was something in the bushes. His reaction in that situation is justified as there is a daily threat of being eaten by a sabretooth.

Way down his lineage is Frank who lives in today's society. Frank works inside all day and has few real safety concerns until one day he is assaulted in a parking lot while walking to his vehicle. Months go by and Frank returns to work, but as soon as he drives into the parking lot he has intense anxiety symptoms. Frank wants to run home and crawl back into bed. Obviously this might make things worse the next time he tries to return to work. Frank could avoid parking lots altogether, maybe even stay inside his safe home for the rest of his life. Again this would cause more problems in the future. Frank sitting in his car with anxiety through the roof decides with his neocortex that it's probably safe to step out of his car and does some deep breathing to lower his heart rate and gain control of his body, next he switches his amygdala off by thinking about how much he appreciates being able to go back to work. With his heart rate lowered and his amygdala silenced Frank can then use his executive functions of foresight and cost benefit analysis and realize that the threat is low and the benefit for him is to return to work. Frank grabs his lunch and leaves his car and some of his anxiety behind as he proceeds on with life.

Operating Yourself with Test Anxiety

What is test anxiety?

I remember sitting down in high school to write my final exams in the gymnasium with hundreds of other students. Even though I studied and felt ready for the test, as soon as we were given the okay to start my mind would draw blank. I couldn't even make sense of the first question. Time would pass and I would start to panic as I fumbled through the first few questions, then slowly as I started answering some of the questions the answers to the others would come back to me, and I would do fine despite the wasted time. This is test anxiety and it happens to a lot of people.

What is happening?

The circumstance of the test was engaging the fear circuitry thus firing the survival system. The amygdala perceived this as a threat and the blood stopped flowing to the top part of my brain where the answers to the test were stored. The blood was redirected to the lower and middle parts of my brain in order to keep me safe from this imagined threat. As I started answering the questions I lowered the fear response and my neocortex reengaged, allowing me access to the answers that were stored in the top part of my brain.

What can you do to manage test anxiety?

Deep breathe to shut off the survival response. Change thinking to reflect thoughts of gratitude, appreciation or love. By asking yourself what is good about this situation, or how good am I going to feel when this test is over is enough to change your thinking. With the fear circuitry turned off and your thoughts focused on the outcome rather than the stress of the moment, you can begin your test. Truthfully, I used to bring a pair of dice with me and roll it with the numerical value corresponding to the letter on the multiple choice section. A few rolls would be enough to interrupt my fear pattern and get me laughing, which engaged the top part of the brain where the answers were.

Operating Yourself with Performance Anxiety

What is performance anxiety?

Public speaking is routinely rated second only to death in polls questioning people's biggest fears. This is because people get performance anxiety. This happens to musicians, actors, public speakers, people in interviews, and many others. When I go to speak to large groups of people, if I focus on remembering my lines, or questioning whether my ankles look fat in these shoes, I trigger the fear response. The amygdala signals that there is a threat and mobilizes the reptilian brain. As the blood stops flowing to the neocortex where my memory has stored my lines, I get more nervous and my mind goes blank. The result is an enhanced fear response and it continues until the fight, flight or freeze response kicks in or we find a way to re-engage the neocortex.

What can you do to manage performance anxiety?

Deep breathe to calm the reptile then change thinking. I usually tell myself that "this is going to be a lot of fun and the audience is going to love this presentation." Or, I focus on appreciating the opportunity to give my message to a new group of people and possibly help people take control of how they operate themselves, which I believe can make a positive impact in people's lives.

Operating Yourself with Depression

Why do people get depression?

Like anxiety, depression has a purpose as it keeps us safe and forces us into a parasympathetic, calming state. A common symptom of depression is sleeping too much because the person with depression wants to lie around with the blanket pulled over their head and hide from the world. If they are overwhelmed, or their filter is over run, depression helps them to go into a dark, quiet space and reset. Depression actually helps people reset their filter by getting them to spend more time in the calming system rather than the activating system. The calming system lets the filter reset and gives their body time to grow, and repair itself.

Another common problem that depressed people encounter is negative thoughts. Often people with depression allow their thoughts to be dominated by the mammalian brain, where logic does not exist. Their emotions pull them around instead of taking control and functioning out of the neocortex.

How can we end depression?

One of the most effective therapies for depression is cognitive behavior therapy or CBT. The success rates of CBT are roughly equal to medication management without the side effects and high relapse rate when treatment concludes. People who do CBT activate a different part of their brain than those who use medication alone to treat depression. A treatment strategy within CBT is called reactivation. Here participants are taught to set behavior goals and take action, which has shown to help people get moving and lead their emotions with their behavior rather than the other way around. In other words, they let the reptile move the mammal back into place through action, instead of sitting around and allowing the mammal to dominate their thinking, which is based on the fear circuitry.

A second CBT strategy that shows effectiveness is cognitive therapy. Cognitive therapy teaches people to recognize their faulty thinking patterns and challenge negative thoughts, replacing them with realistic thoughts that then improve mood. Thus, teaching people to activate their neocortex and take control of their thoughts to create a positive neuromap by changing their thinking habits.

Operating Yourself with Anger

What contributes to anger?

When we start to get angry our survival mechanisms mobilize and the blood begins to flow to the middle and lower parts of the brain. The more activated we become, the more likely we do something that we will later regret. Anger isn't all bad. It can be a warning sign that something is wrong and we need to pay attention so we can correct our course, however most people don't heed the warning signal. Ignoring the warning can cause us to function solely out of the mammalian brain, by passing the neocortex, the logic center. We react to the environment instead of consciously choosing our actions. Operating from the mammalian brain is why we do things when angry that we later regret we aren't operating our self from our place of higher thought.

What can you do to manage anger?

Start by paying attention to the warning signs. Each of us experience physical sensations that are associated with anger. Heeding these can help us identify that we are increasing our anger state. When we are in the yellow or caution zone catch the anger before we move into the red or danger zone. The earlier we detect and do something about it the easier it is to take control. Again, deep breathe to turn the reptile off, and replace your thoughts with those of appreciation, gratitude or love to shut down the amygdala. Next, do something to deal with the anger. If you are angry at a certain person and it's safe to talk to them about it, do it before your anger returns. Use the mobilizing power of anger to your advantage before it's so strong that it over rides your conscious thoughts and you find yourself reacting from it instead of harnessing its power to work for you. Take charge of your anger and speak up assertively, not aggressively. You may be surprised with the results.

Warranty

You are the only you, you have. Look after yourself. You can't trade yourself in, or return yourself to Walmart to get a new you. Accept yourself. If you have a defect such as a hideous mole under your right eye and are unwilling to pay a small fortune to have someone burn it off with a laser, accept it. It's a part of you, and you are an amazing being who is capable of incredible acts of you-ness. Remember, what any human can do, to a certain extent, you can do. Embrace your awesomeness. Unleash your individuality and allow yourself to be spectacular, because you are, despite what others who may be afraid of unleashing their own spectacular-ness may say. They only say it because of their own fear. They are scared into place, and the mere thought of setting down their fears and living an amazing life, causes so much internal panic that they devote more time holding themselves back, and also holding others around them back, too. Don't listen. Live spectacular, I dare you. You're the only you, you have. Unleash the awesome!

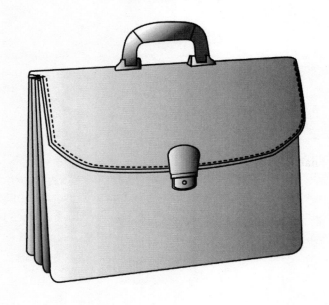

Don't forget your briefcase!

Glossary

Mammalian: the mammalian brain operates our basic emotions, memory, and motivation. It is where emotion and physical sensations are attached to memory. At this level, emotions are simply the chemical communication signals that get converted into physical sensations, which our conscious mind identifies as emotions. The mammalian brain also houses our reward and fear pathways giving us pleasure and pain.

Neocortex: the neo-cortex, which simply translates into "neo" meaning "new" and "cortex" meaning "brain," thus new brain. This is the last part to develop and is essentially responsible for making us human and giving us the control panel of human functioning. This is the part that gives us language, creativity, abstract thought, and the ability to think logically and make conscious decisions.

Neuromap: a neuromap is basically a cluster of connections, organized around a certain event, behavior, thought, or feelings. Its purpose is to increase efficiency and decrease energy output when doing repetitive things. This is the basis of habit formation and why we have that feeling of automatic pilot after doing something we have done 791 times before.

Neuroplasticity: neuroplasticity refers to the brains ability to change, reorganize and rewire itself. Previously, scientists believed that the brain didn't change after a specific age but now they know that the brain is able to change. The brain is malleable or plastic.

Reptilian: the reptilian brain operates at the most basic level of survival. It includes the functions of respiration, digestion, circulation, and reproduction. This is the most primitive and instinctual part of our brain.

Reading List

Evolve your Brain, Joe Dispenza, D.C.

Why Zebras Don't Get Ulcers, Robert M. Sapolsky

Change Your Brain, Change Your Life, Daniel G. Amen, M.D.

The Owner's Manual for The Brain, Pierce J. Howard, Ph.D.

What Happy People Know, Dan Baker, Ph.D.

My Stroke of Insight, Jill Bolte Taylor, Ph.D.

Brain Rules, John Medina

The Brain That Changes Itself, Norman Doidge, M.D.

Biology of Belief, Bruce Lipton, Ph.D.